WHERE TO LAUNCH AROUND THE COAST

Where to Launch Around the Coast

Compiled by

Diana van der Klugt

Opus Book Publishing Limited

Acknowledgements
The Publishers would like to thank the many Harbour Masters, Local Authorities,
Agencies and individuals who have helped to update the 5th edition of this book

First Published 1986
New Editions 1988, 1990, 1994, 2000

ISBN 1-898574-05-7

Copyright © Opus Book Publishing Ltd
Millhouse, Riseden Road, Wadhurst, East Sussex

Whilst every care has been taken in the compilation of this guide, no responsibility
can be taken for the existence of any inaccuracies contained in the information
published in this book. A reference to any particular site in this book is not evidence
of a right of way to the site or of public availability at any time and the inclusion of any
slipway in this book cannot be taken as a recommendation of such a site. The publishers
do not hold themselves responsible for any accident which arises as a result of any
site mentioned in this book being used.

Cover Design: Dave Steele Mac Services

Printed by Biddles Ltd
Woodbridge Park Estate, Guildford

Contents

INTRODUCTION

Trail-boats come in many shapes and sizes, from small sailing dinghies to larger powerboats, but they require much the same facility - a good launching site or slipway, to enable them to be put to their proper water-borne use as quickly as possible. They are used by many different types of watersports enthusiasts - wind-surfers, water-skiers, dinghy sailors, divers, fishermen, trailer-sailors and especially weekend potterers who live miles from the sea but get enjoyment from visiting different coastal areas. But a good slipway must be able to offer other facilities, in particular parking for car and trailer, and useful amenities such as toilets, fuel or chandlery. All this information and much more, will be found for over 700 sites in the latest edition of the popular guide WHERE TO LAUNCH AROUND THE COAST.

Using The Book

The book is divided geographically into seven sections, starting with the West Country and then following an anti-clockwise direction around the British Coast: each section is prefaced by a sketch map of the area covered showing the location of the majority of sites and there is also a comprehensive index at the end of the book to facilitate quick reference to a particular site. Where possible, the following details are given for each site:

Name of site and contact telephone number of owner/controlling authority (where applicable)

Type:	*construction and equipment*
Suits:	*recommended craft type and size*
Availability:	*tidal access or other time constraints*
Restrictions:	*speed limits in force, local dangers, prohibition of certain types of craft, restricting factors for access*
Facilities:	*availability of fuel, parking for car and trailer, toilets and showers, chandlery, diving supplies, outboard repairs etc: (c) indicates a charge for the facility*
Dues:	*any harbour or local dues payable*
Charge:	*launching fee, if applicable; charges quoted are for launching and retrieving a 15'/4.6m LOA boat unless otherwise stated*
Directions:	*directions from the nearest main road plus local directions*
Waters accessed:	*the local bay, estuary, loch or general sea area accessed by the slipway*

7

Most sites described are suitable for craft up to 18'/5.5m length over all (LOA) unless specified. A site described as suitable for dinghies only, usually has restricted access which may mean that the boat has to be manhandled into the water. The hours of availability given for coastal sites are intended as a guide only; obviously this is a matter that depends very much on the type of craft to be launched and on the conditions prevailing at the time. In the case of larger craft, especially those with a deep draught, launching should be undertaken as near high water (HW) as possible although at some exposed sites, sea conditions at high water can be dangerous. Many sites can be used to launch smaller craft at most states of tide, especially if the trailer can be manhandled across the beach to the water.

Before launching you should always make sure that you are aware of any local restrictions or bye-laws which may be in force. This particularly applies to those wishing to launch powerboats and pwc or to water-ski. In many popular bathing areas, these activities are restricted to clearly defined areas and there are heavy penalties for infringement of the bye-laws; those wishing to water-ski should always be aware of the danger which can be present to bathers. In an increasing number of areas, craft wishing to launch must be able to produce evidenbce of 3rd party insurance cover. In many harbours, especially those on the South Coast harbour dues are charged. Where possible, it is advisable to contact the owner or authority in charge of a site before setting out to establish the suitability of a site for your purposes.

Throughout the book, the following abbreviations have been used:

HW	high water
LW	low water
S	spring tides
N	neap tides
HWS	high water springs
LWS	low water springs
pwc	personal water craft
Hb Mr	Harbour Master
T.I.C.	Tourist Information Centre
hp	horse power
inc.	including
BH	Bank Holiday
(c)	indicates that there is a charge

Safety

When putting to sea for however long or far, precautions must be taken and certain equipment carried. Remember the following:

1. Know the limitations of your craft
2. Learn the "Rules of the Road" and be aware of any local bye-laws regarding speed limits, use of craft, prohibitions on certain activities etc.
3. Seek local knowledge or talk to the Coastguard, who can warn of local dangers
4. Inform someone of where you are going and how long you expect to be away
5. Listen to local weather forecasts and heed any warnings of adverse weather

All craft should carry:

1. A means of sound signalling, and navigation lights, if used between sunset and sunrise
2. An extra means of propulsion, if only oars or paddles
3. An anchor and plenty of line
4. A suitable bailer
5. Lifejackets or buoyancy aids for all the crew, preferably to be worn at all times
6. Warm and waterproof clothing
7. Flares: two red hand flares and two orange smoke signals for small craft
8. Local charts, tide tables and a compass

TRAILERS AND THE LAW

The trailer is very often the neglected part of the boating package. Whilst hulls, engines and other equipment are well-maintained the trailer lies idly by, in the open, unprotected and usually without a squirt of grease. The moment the sun appears, however, it is hitched up with its load and expected to perform perfectly in delivering its charge to the water's edge. Do give it a chance! Protect those bearings with grease and put a dab on the ballhitch. Check the tyres and lights and above all make sure it is legal. Our trailer laws have been brought into line with other EEC countries and you must conform, otherwise you risk your weekend or holiday being marred by a brush with the police.

Towing Speeds

These are 60 mph on motorways and dual carriageways and 50 mph on other roads, provided no lower limit is in force. Vehicles towing trailers are not allowed in the third lane of a motorway.

Braking Regulations

If brakes are fitted to a trailer they must be in working order, even on trailers where brakes are not compulsory.

Trailers without brakes
You may use an unbraked trailer with a gross weight (total of trailer, boat and contents) of up to 750kg (15cwt), provided the towing vehicle's kerbside weight is at least twice the gross weight of the trailer. It should be remembered that towing an unbraked trailer of the max. legal weight can increase your safe stopping distance.

Overrun braked trailers
The max. gross weight (total of trailer, boat and contents) must not exceed 3500kg. Vehicle manufacturers generally recommend the max. towing weight for each model: this is not the legal max. but a measure of the vehicle's ability to tow. As a rule of thumb, do not exceed 85% of the kerbside weight of the towing vehicle.

Trailer dimensions

The maximum width of a trailer when being towed by a motor car or light goods vehicle is 2.3m. In all other cases (HGV) this is 2.5m. The trailer load must not extend more than 305mm outwards on either side of the towing vehicle. The maximum load width allowable, without police advice and supervision, is 2.9m. A trailer and its load must not normally exceed 7m in length excluding drawbar and coupling.

Lighting Regulations

Two red tail lights and brake lights must be fitted which operate with the towing vehicle lights. Two amber indicators must flash in unison with the towing vehicle indicators. Two red triangular reflectors of the approved type must be fitted to the rear of the trailer and the number plate area must be illuminated. Trailers exceeding 5m in length must also be fitted with orange side-facing reflectors.

This is only a brief outline of the law affecting trailers and we advise anyone who intends to trail their boat to check on the current regulations in force.

Indespension publish the "Indespension Trailer Manual", an invaluable guide to trailers and towing. The 10th edition has been re-written to reflect the needs and legislation of the late 1990s and can be obtained from the company.
Contact: Indespension Ltd, Belmont Road, Bolton BL1 7AQ, Tel: (01204) 309797 Fax: (01204) 596928.

ENVIRONMENT AGENCY

The Environment Agency is the Inland Navigation Authority for 800km of river, estuaries and harbours in England and Wales. It aims to maintain and manage these navigations to a high standard for the enjoyment and safety of the boater. The waterways under the Agency's management contrast greatly, from remote Fenland rivers and the upper reaches of the Thames, to the grandeur of the lower Thames, and the commercial Harbour of Rye.

Work carried out by the Environment Agency includes maintaining and operating locks, dredging, licensing boats, enforcing speed limits and providing amenities that directly improve navigations. These include moorings, toilet and sanitation facilities.

The Agency has a key role in providing information to boat owners and users of the rivers to enhance their recreation potential.

The Environment Agency also works to improve water quality, fisheries, recreation and conservation on all its navigations. This is done to enhance your enjoyment of the water environment, be you afloat or on the bank. The river corridors, estuaries and harbours also provide important habitats for many types of animal and plant.

For further information on the Agency's roles and any information on licensing contact:

Environment Agency
Rio House
Waterside Drive, Aztec West
Almondsbury
Bristol
BS32 4UD

Tel: 01454 624400

CLEAN SEAS

Remember - it is illegal to dispose of garbage, plastic, waste oil, sewage or any toxic substance at sea. Please bring your waste ashore and dispose of it responsibly.

British Marine Industry Federation (BMIF),
Meadlake Place,Thorpe Lea Road, Egham, Surrey TW20 8HE.
Tel: (01784) 472222

British Disabled Water Ski Federation,
Heron Lake, Hythe End, Wraysbury, Middlesex, TW19 6HW.
Tel: (01784) 483664

British Water Ski Federation,
390 City Road, London, EC1V 2QA.
Tel: (020) 7833 2855

British Waterways
Willow Grange, Church Road, Watford WD1 3QA
Tel: (01923) 226422 Fax: (01923) 201400

Broads Authority,
Thomas Harvey House, 18 Colegate, Norwich, Norfolk, NR3 1BQ.
Tel: (01603) 610734

Dinghy Cruising Association,
56 Grebe Crescent, Horsham, West Sussex RH13 6ED
Tel: (01403) 266800

Environment Agency,
Rio House, Waterside Drive, Aztec West,Almondsbury,
Bristol, BS32 4UD Tel: (01454) 624400 Fax: (01454) 624409

HM Coastguard,
Spring Place, 105 Commercial Road, Southampton,
Hants, SO15 1EG. Tel: (023) 8032 9100 Fax: (023) 8032 9488

Hydrographic Office,
Taunton, Somerset. TA1 2DN, Tel: (01823) 337900

Meteorological Office,
London Road, Bracknell, Berks, RG12 2SY. Tel: (01344) 856655

National Federation of Sea Schools,
Staddlestones, Fletchwood Lane, Totton, Southampton,
Hants, SO4 2DZ Tel: (023) 8029 3822 Fax: (023) 8029 3822

Port of London Authority,
Devon House, St Katherine's Way, London EC1 9LB.
Tel: (020) 7265 2656

Royal Institute of Navigation,
1 Kensington Gore, London SW7 2A, Tel: (020) 7589 5021

Royal National Lifeboat Institution,
West Quay Road, Poole, Dorset, BH15 1HZ
Tel: (01202) 663000 Fax: (01202) 663167

Royal Yachting Association,
RYA House, Romsey Road, Eastleigh, Hants. SO50 9YA
Tel: (020) 8062 7400 Fax: (020) 8062 9924

Trail Sail Association,
Scape Haven, 22 Grand Stand, Scapegoat Hill, Golcar,
Huddersfield, HD7 4NQ Tel: (01532) 533616

Trinity House,
Trinity Square, Tower Hill, London, EC3N 4DH.
Tel: (020) 7480 6601

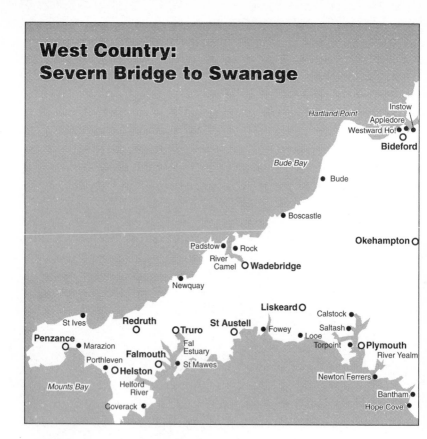

West Country: Severn Bridge to Swanage

Beachley Point - Car Ferry Slipway, Ferry Road

Type:	stone slipway under Severn Bridge
Suits:	small powered craft only: no sailing craft
Availability:	at all times except LWS
Restrictions:	12 knot speed limit (except designated areas): site is subject to fierce tidal currents (up to 12 knots) across the slip and is only suitable for experienced boaters with adequately powered craft
Facilities:	fuel (3 miles), limited parking for car and trailer nearby, toilets in pub
Dues:	none
Charge:	none
Directions:	take A48 from Chepstow towards Gloucester, turning right after 1 mile following signs to Sedbury and Beachley: site is at end of road
Waters accessed:	Severn Estuary and Bristol Channel

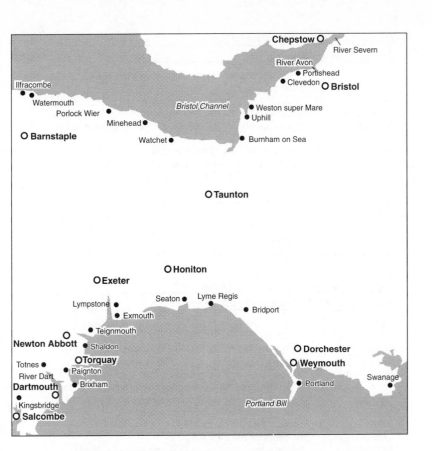

Lydney Docks - Lydney Yacht Club, Harbour Road

Tel: (01989) 750396

Type:	steep concrete ramp
Suits:	sailing craft with additional power
Availability:	approx. 1 hour either side HW with prior permission of Yacht Club
Restrictions:	12 knot speed limit (except in designated areas): site is subject to fierce tidal currents (up to 12 knots) and is only suitable for experienced boaters with adequately prepared craft; access is via a narrow unmetalled road and club compound has locked gate
Facilities:	fuel in Lydney, limited parking for car and trailer, toilets and clubhouse with bar
Dues:	none
Charge:	approx. £5
Directions:	from A48 Lydney by-pass follow signs to the railway station, then continue along Harbour Road to Lydney Docks
Waters accessed:	Severn Estuary and Bristol Channel

Bristol - Bristol Marina, Hanover Place
Tel: (0117) 926 5730

Type:	wide concrete ramp into deep water of Floating Harbour
Suits:	all craft up to approx. 18'/5.5m LOA
Availability:	all states of tide 0900-2200
Restrictions:	6 mph speed limit in harbour; all craft must have navigation licence
Facilities:	diesel on site, petrol nearby, parking for car and trailer, toilets, chandlery and full marina facilities on site
Dues:	approx £5.60 for 24hr licence (available from marina office)
Charge:	no separate fee charged
Directions:	from city centre follow signs to "SS Great Britain" and Historic Harbour: access is via Cumberland Rd and Hanover Place
Waters accessed:	Severn Estuary, Bristol Channel and Kennet and Avon Canal

Bristol - Underfall Yard, Cumberland Road
Tel: (0117) 903 1484 (Harbour Office)

Type:	concrete slipway into min 3'/1m water in Floating Harbour
Suits:	all craft up to 18'/5.5m LOA
Availability:	0800 -1700 (winter), 0800 - dusk (summer)
Restrictions:	6 mph speed limit in harbour, 4 mph in canal and river: water-skiing permitted at certain times, pwc prohibited
Facilities:	fuel nearby, parking for car and trailer on site, toilets, chandlery and outboard repairs nearby
Dues:	approx. £4.20
Charge:	no separate fee charged
Directions:	follow signs to dock area from city centre: access is via Cumberland Rd and through Underfall Yard
Waters accessed:	River Avon, Severn Estuary and Bristol Channel

Portishead - Portishead Quays Marina
Tel: (02920) 705021

Type:	35 ton travel hoist
Suits:	larger craft
Availability:	approx. 2 hours either side HW from 0900-1730 by prior arrangement
Restrictions:	none
Facilities:	fuel nearby, parking for car and trailer and toilets on site, boat storage in locked compound: full marina facilities and boating lake for sailing dinghies available Spring 2001
Dues:	none
Charge:	approx. £8.50 per metre
Directions:	leave M5 at junction 19 and follow signs to Portishead: follow road through town and turn right into Harbour Rd, then take first left
Waters accessed:	Bristol Channel

Clevedon - Clevedon Slipway, Seafront

Tel: (01934) 634994/3 (Seafront Officer)

Type:	steep concrete slipway with narrow entrance
Suits:	dinghies and small powered craft: no pwc
Availability:	approx. 2 hours either side HW
Restrictions:	speed limit inshore: water-skiing permitted offshore; no pwc
Facilities:	fuel in town, parking for car and toilets nearby
Dues:	none
Charge:	none
Directions:	leave M5 at junction 20: site is 50m west of pier
Waters accessed:	Severn Estuary and Bristol Channel

Weston-super-Mare - Knightstone Slipway, Marine Parade

Tel: (01934) 634994/3 (Seafront Officer)

Type:	wide concrete slipway
Suits:	all craft except pwc
Availability:	approx. 2 hours either side HW by prior arrangement
Restrictions:	5 mph speed limit in harbour between pier and Knightstone Point: no water-skiing in this area; contact local water-ski club: no pwc
Facilities:	fuel in town, parking for car nearby, toilets, chandlery and outboard repairs all nearby
Dues:	none
Charge:	none
Directions:	leave M5 at junction 21 and take A370 to town centre, turning right at seafront: site is at north end of town near Knightstone Point and Marina Lake
Waters accessed:	Severn Estuary and Bristol Channel

Weston-super-Mare - Uphill Boat Centre, Uphill Wharf

Tel: (01934) 418617

Type:	medium concrete ramp
Suits:	all craft up to 45'/13m LOA
Availability:	approx. 2 hours either side HW from 0700 - 2100
Restrictions:	6 knot speed limit in river: water-skiing permitted in Weston Bay
Facilities:	diesel on site, petrol nearby, parking for car and trailer, toilets and showers, chandlery, outboard repairs, moorings and accommodation all available on site: marine lake for windsurfing and canoeing
Dues:	none
Charge:	approx. £5
Directions:	follow signs to 'Uphill Beach and Sands' from M5
Waters accessed:	River Axe, Weston Bay and Bristol Channel

Burnham-on-Sea - South Esplanade

Tel: (01278) 787852 (Tourist Information Centre)

Type:	concrete and wooden slipway with 15cwt weight limit
Suits:	small powered and sailing craft
Availability:	approx. 2 hours either side HW: at LW currents are strong and there is a lot of mud
Restrictions:	8 knot speed limit: water-skiing permitted in designated area; pwc must be used safely; narrow slipway gets very congested
Facilities:	fuel nearby, parking for car (c) nearby and trailer (sometimes) on site, toilets
Dues:	none
Charge:	none: but permit required to use slipway is obtainable free from Tourist Information Centre (see number above)
Directions:	leave M5 at junction 22 following signs to Burnham-on-Sea: site is at south end of Esplanade at the end of Pier St
Waters accessed:	Rivers Parrett and Brue, Bridgwater Bay and Bristol Channel

Watchet - Harbour Slipway

Tel: (01984) 631264 (Harbour Master)

Type:	concrete slipway
Suits:	all craft up to 30'/9m LOA
Availability:	approx. 3 hours either side HW
Restrictions:	5 mph speed limit: narrow access road: a marina is to be built here which may affect the slipway - tel. Hb Mr for latest information
Facilities:	fuel (2 miles), parking for car and trailer in Market St (c), toilets and chandlery nearby; local Boat Owners Assoc. has compound and welcomes visitors
Dues:	none
Charge:	approx. £1.25
Directions:	follow A39 from Bridgwater or A358 from Taunton to Williton, turning off to Watchet
Waters accessed:	Bristol Channel

Minehead - Harbour Slipway

Tel: (01643) 702566/707651 (Harbour Master)

Type:	shallow concrete ramp onto sand
Suits:	craft up to 30'/9m LOA except pwc
Availability:	approx. 2½ hours either side HW by prior arrangement
Restrictions:	3 mph speed limit in harbour: pwc prohibited. **Caution:** overhead telephone wire adjacent to slipway
Facilities:	fuel (½ mile), parking for car and trailer nearby (c), toilets nearby; pub, cafe and tackle shop on quay; local sailing club has compound and welcomes visitors
Dues:	none
Charge:	approx. £1.70
Directions:	follow A358 from Taunton to Williton then the A39
Waters accessed:	Bristol Channel

Watermouth - Watermouth Harbour

Tel: (01271) 865422 (Harbour Master)

Type:	concrete slipway onto hard sand
Suits:	all craft
Availability:	all states of tide for dinghies, near HW for larger craft
Restrictions:	3 knot speed limit in harbour, water-skiing permitted outside harbour; slipway is used to launch Lifeboat and must be kept clear at all times
Facilities:	fuel, parking for car and trailer nearby, visitor's moorings
Dues:	none
Charge:	approx. £3
Directions:	from Barnstaple follow A39 and B3229 north then A399 west: harbour is 4 miles east of Ilfracombe, opposite Watermouth Castle
Waters accessed:	Bristol Channel

Ilfracombe - Harbour Slipway

Tel: (01271) 862108 (Harbour Master - Summer only)

Type:	shallow concrete ramp onto hard sand
Suits:	all craft up to approx. 18'/5.5m LOA
Availability:	approx. 3 hours either side HW: access gates are closed when tides are over 31'/9.6m high
Restrictions:	4 knot speed limit in harbour: pwc, windsurfers and water-skiing prohibited; contact the Harbour Master before use in summer; slipway is used to launch Lifeboat and must be kept clear at all times
Facilities:	diesel on site, petrol nearby, parking for car and trailer (c) and toilets on site
Dues:	none
Charge:	none
Directions:	from Barnstaple follow A361 or signs from Blackmoor Gate
Waters accessed:	Bristol Channel

Instow (River Torridge) - Instow Promenade

Tel: (01271) 861081 (Instow Marine Services - Harbour Master)

Type:	concrete slipway onto sand
Suits:	small craft
Availability:	approx. 3 hours either side HW
Restrictions:	7 knot speed limit in estuary; water-skiing in designated area
Facilities:	diesel, parking for car and trailer (c), crane and assistance with launching, outboard repairs on site; chandlery and diving supplies in Bideford
Dues:	none
Charge:	none
Directions:	from Barnstaple/Bideford follow A39: site is off road on east side of River Torridge
Waters accessed:	Taw and Torridge Estuaries and Bristol Channel

Bideford (River Torridge) - Bank End Slipway
Tel: (01237) 477676 (Tourist Information Centre, Victoria Park)

Type:	concrete slipway onto soft mud and sand
Suits:	small craft
Availability:	1½ hours either side HW
Restrictions:	7 knot speed limit in estuary: water-skiing in designated area
Facilities:	fuel from garage (200m), parking for car and trailer on site (c), toilets in Victoria Park (100m), chandlery and diving supplies in Bideford
Dues:	none
Charge:	none
Directions:	follow A39 west from Barnstaple, turning left after crossing river: site is adjacent to Bideford Quay with access through car park
Waters accessed:	River Torridge and Bristol Channel

Appledore (River Torridge) - Churchfields Slipway

Type:	concrete slipway onto shingle beach
Suits:	all craft
Availability:	approx. 5 hours either side HW
Restrictions:	7 knot speed limit in estuary: water-skiing in designated area
Facilities:	fuel nearby, parking for car and trailer on site (c), toilets (50m), chandlery and diving supplies from Bideford
Dues:	none
Charge:	none
Directions:	follow A39 to outskirts of Bideford: at Heywood Road roundabout take the A386 to Appledore; site is in Churchfields Car Park at end of quay
Waters accessed:	River Torridge and Bristol Channel

Westward Ho! - Slipway, Westbourne Terrace

Type:	concrete slipway onto sand
Suits:	small craft which can be manhandled only
Availability:	at all states of tide but launching may be difficult at HW due to heavy breaking seas
Restrictions:	7 knot speed limit in certain areas: before launching craft must be manhandled over large sandy beach
Facilities:	parking for car and trailer on site (c), toilets in Golf Links Road (100m), chandlery and diving supplies from Bideford
Dues:	none
Charge:	none
Directions:	follow A39 to Bideford outskirts taking B3236 to Westward Ho! town centre: site is at end of Westbourne Terrace
Waters accessed:	Barnstaple Bay and Bristol Channel

Bude - Harbour Slipway
Tel: (01288) 353111 (Harbour Master)

Type:	steep stone and concrete slipway
Suits:	all craft
Availability:	approx. 2 hours either side HW
Restrictions:	access is via a narrow road along the breakwater: pwc are prohibited from this site and water-skiing is only permitted offshore; the use of this site is very dependent on sea and weather conditions - consult the Harbour Master before launching
Facilities:	fuel from garages in town, parking for car and trailer nearby (c 1st Apr-30th Sept), toilets nearby
Dues:	none
Charge:	approx. £25 p.a.
Directions:	follow A39 south from Barnstaple or B3254/A3072 north from Launceston: site is near sea lock at entrance to Bude Canal
Waters accessed:	Bude Bay

Boscastle Harbour - Harbour Slip
Tel: (01840) 250453 (Harbour Master)

Type:	shallow concrete slipway
Suits:	small powered craft and trailer-sailers: no pwc
Availability:	approx. 1½ hours either side HW with Hbr Mr's permission
Restrictions:	3 knot speed limit in harbour: windsurfers and pwc prohibited
Facilities:	fuel nearby, parking for car in car park nearby (c) but trailers can be left in the boat park, toilets
Dues:	none
Charge:	approx. £3 (weekly rates available)
Directions:	turn off the A39 onto the B3263: site is at head of harbour
Waters accessed:	Atlantic Ocean

Rock (River Camel) - The Quay, Rock Sailing & Waterski Club
Tel: (01208) 862709

Type:	shallow concrete ramp onto sandy beach
Suits:	all craft except pwc
Availability:	approx. 2 hours either side HW
Restrictions:	8 knot speed limit in moorings: water-skiing permitted in designated areas upstream but pwc prohibited; no parking on beach or slipway; site is busy in season
Facilities:	fuel, parking for car and trailer, toilets and outboard repairs nearby
Dues:	approx. £3.50 (£15 per week)
Charge:	no separate fee charged
Directions:	from Bideford follow A39 to Wadebridge, turning onto B3314 then following minor roads to Rock
Waters accessed:	Camel Estuary and Padstow Bay

Rock (River Camel) - Ferry Point Slip
Tel: (01841) 532239 (Harbour Office)

Type:	shallow concrete ramp onto sandy beach
Suits:	small craft except pwc
Availability:	at all states of tide
Restrictions:	8 knot speed limit: water-skiing permitted in designated area but pwc prohibited; no vehicles to park in dinghy park
Facilities:	fuel nearby, parking for car nearby (c) and for trailer on site, toilets, chandlery and outboard repairs nearby
Dues:	approx. £3.50 (under 10hp) or £5 (over 10hp)
Charge:	no separate fee charged
Directions:	from Bideford follow A39 to Wadebridge, turning onto B3314 then following minor roads to Rock: access to site is through car park
Waters accessed:	Camel Estuary and Padstow Bay

Wadebridge (River Camel) - The Quay, off Eddystone Road
Tel: (01841) 532239 (Harbour Office)

Type:	shallow concrete ramp
Suits:	small powered craft except pwc
Availability:	approx. 3 hours either side HW by prior arrangement
Restrictions:	8 knot speed limit; water-skiing, windsurfing and pwc prohibited
Facilities:	fuel in town, parking for car nearby (c), outboard repairs nearby
Dues:	approx. £3.50 (under 10hp) or £5 (over 10hp)
Charge:	no separate fee charged
Directions:	from Bideford or Bude follow A39 into town: cross the bridge to south side of estuary and turn right into Eddystone Rd: site is on quay after about 350m
Waters accessed:	Camel Estuary and Padstow Bay

Wadebridge (River Camel) - Trevilling Quay Road (Chapman and Hewitt)
Tel: (01208) 813487

Type:	concrete slipway
Suits:	all craft
Availability:	approx. 2 hours either side HW by prior arrangement
Restrictions:	5 knot speed limit; water-skiing permitted in designated areas
Facilities:	diesel, parking for car and trailer (c), chandlery, crane hire and all boatyard facilities available on site
Dues:	approx. £3.50 (under 10hp) or £5 (over 10hp))
Charge:	approx. £18
Directions:	from Bideford or Bude follow A39 into town: site is on north side of estuary
Waters accessed:	Camel Estuary and Padstow Bay

Padstow (Camel Estuary) - Sailing Club Slip (South Slip), West Quay
Tel: (01841) 532239 (Harbour Office)

Type:	steep and fairly narrow concrete slipway
Suits:	all craft up to approx. 17'/5m LOA
Availability:	approx. 3 hours either side HW
Restrictions:	8 knot speed limit: water-skiing is permitted in designated area upstream and pwc are regulated
Facilities:	diesel on site, petrol nearby, parking for car and trailer (c) and toilets on site: chandlery and outboard repairs nearby
Dues:	approx £3.50 (under 10hp) or £5 (over 10hp): pwc £40
Charge:	no additional fee charged
Directions:	follow A39 from Bideford, then A389 west of Wadebridge: site is adjacent Harbour Office and access is through car park
Waters accessed:	Camel Estuary and Padstow Bay

Newquay - Harbour Slip, South Quay Hill
Tel (01637) 872809 (Harbour Master)

Type:	shallow granite slipway onto beach
Suits:	all craft except pwc
Availability:	approx. 4 hours either side HW
Restrictions:	4 knot speed limit in and out of harbour: water-skiing allowed 400m off beaches but pwc are prohibited; 4-wheel drive vehicles are recommended for launching over beach and breaking waves can prevent launching; all boats should carry safety equipment and a safety briefing from the Harbour Master is required
Facilities:	diesel, limited parking for car and trailer (c), toilets, chandlery and diving supplies all on site: boats cannot be left overnight
Dues:	none
Charge:	approx. £2.50
Directions:	from A39 Bideford road take A3059, or A3058 from A30: site is NE of town and access is via narrow and steep road; access can be very congested in summer
Waters accessed:	Newquay Bay and Watergate Bay

St Ives - Old Lifeboat Slipway, Wharf Road
Tel: (01736) 795018 (Harbour Master)

Type:	shallow concrete ramp onto hard sandy beach
Suits:	all craft except pwc
Availability:	approx 2½ hours either side HW from ramp
Restrictions:	5 mph speed limit ; no water-skiing or pwc in harbour; concrete slip must be kept clear at all times: contact Harbour Master prior to use
Facilities:	petrol, parking for car and trailer (c), toilets and chandlery all nearby
Dues:	approx. £9.70: pwc £27
Charge:	no additional fee charged
Directions:	take A3074 off A30 Penzance road; slipway is adjacent to the main road through the town
Waters accessed:	St Ives Bay

Penzance Harbour - Albert Pier Slipway
Tel (01736) 366113 (Harbour Office, Wharf Road)

Type:	concrete slipway
Suits:	all craft
Availability:	2-3 hours either side HW
Restrictions:	5 knot speed limit in harbour: water-skiing allowed offshore; pwc permitted provided speed limit in harbour is observed
Facilities:	diesel on site, petrol nearby, parking for car and trailer on site (c), toilets, chandlery and outboard repairs available nearby
Dues:	approx. £5
Charge:	none
Directions:	follow A30 into town, going past BR station then turning left past the Bus Station and site is 100m on right by the sailing club
Waters accessed:	Mounts Bay

Marazion

Type:	concrete slipway onto sandy beach
Suits:	small craft which can be manhandled
Availability:	most states of tide
Restrictions:	speed limit
Facilities:	fuel nearby, parking for car and trailer (c), toilets in village
Dues:	none
Charge:	none
Directions:	from Penzance follow A30 east: site is close to causeway to St Michaels Mount
Waters accessed:	Mounts Bay

Porthleven - Quayside
Tel (01326) 574270 (Harbour Master)

Type:	concrete slipway
Suits:	all craft
Availability:	approx. 3 hours either side HW
Restrictions:	3 mph speed limit in Inner Harbour, 5 mph in Outer Harbour: no water-skiing; harbour is primarily a fishing harbour and exposed in strong S to SW winds when launching is not permitted
Facilities:	fuel nearby, parking for car and trailer in nearby car park (c), toilets and chandlery nearby, other facilities in Falmouth
Dues:	included in launching fee
Charge:	on application to Harbour Master
Directions:	turn off A394 at Helston then take B3304 for 2 miles to Portleven
Waters accessed:	Mounts Bay

Coverack - Harbour Slipway

Tel: (01326) 280545 (Harbour Master)

Type:	steep concrete ramp onto firm sand
Suits:	sailing dinghies, windsurfers and canoes: no powered craft
Availability:	approx. 2-3 hours either side HW by arrangement with Hbr Mr
Restrictions:	speed limit inshore: pwc and powered craft prohibited in harbour; site is sheltered in SW winds
Facilities:	fuel nearby, parking for car and trailer and toilets nearby
Dues:	approx £3
Charge:	approx. £3
Directions:	turn off A394 at Helston, taking the A3083 and then B3293/3294: site is on east side of Lizard Peninsula: access is via narrow road through village
Waters accessed:	English Channel east of Lizard Peninsula

Falmouth Bay is a designated Special Area of Conservation - all users of the area should respect the environment and not cause pollution

Gillan Creek - St Anthony-in-Meneage

Tel: (01326) 231357 (Sailaway St Anthony Ltd)

Type:	shingle foreshore
Suits:	craft up to 24'/7m LOA except pwc and dive voats
Availability:	approx. 3 hours either side HW from 0800-1800 by prior arrangement
Restrictions:	6 knot speed limit in creek: dive boats and pwc prohibited; access roads are narrow and steep
Facilities:	diesel, parking for car and trailer (c),toilets, chandlery, moorings, boat park and repairs all on site; tractor assistance available during working hours
Dues:	none
Charge:	approx. £4
Directions:	from Helston take the A3083 then B3293 for St Keverne: turn left before Goonhilly Satellite Station for Helford then follow signs for St Anthony
Waters accessed:	Helford River and Falmouth Bay

Gweek (Helford River) - Gweek Quay Boatyard

Tel: (01326) 221657

Type:	medium to shallow concrete ramp
Suits:	all craft with draught up to 9'/2.7m: crane to 40 tons
Availability:	approx. 2 hours either side HW 0900-1800 by prior arrangement
Restrictions:	6 knot speed limit in river: water-skiing prohibited
Facilities:	diesel on site, petrol nearby, parking for car and trailer on site (c if longer than 1 week), toilets & shower, chandlery, moorings, cafe and all yard facilities on site, pub nearby
Dues:	approx. £1.50 per m per week
Charge:	approx. £10
Directions:	from Helston, follow signs to the Lizard and St Keverne or the 'Seal Sanctuary', then to Gweek
Waters accessed:	Helford River and Falmouth Bay

Helford River - Port Navas

Type:	launching over hard shingle foreshore
Suits:	small craft only
Availability:	approx. 2-3 hours either side HW
Restrictions:	6 knot speed limit in river: water-skiing prohibited; narrow and limited access
Facilities:	very limited parking for car and trailer nearby, Port Navas Y.C. nearby
Dues:	none
Charge:	none
Directions:	from A394 (Penryn to Helston road) turn off in Mabe Burnthouse following signs to Mawnan Smith, then Constantine and Port Navas; site is at head of creek
Waters accessed:	Helford River and Falmouth Bay

Helford River - Helford Passage (opposite Ferry Boat Inn)

Tel: (01326) 250625 (Ferry Boat Inn)

Type:	launching over hard shingle foreshore
Suits:	craft up to 18'/5.5m LOA
Availability:	approx. 4 hours either side HW
Restrictions:	no vehicle access to site - launching only with permission of site owner (Ferry Boat Inn Tel: (01326) 250625): 6 knot speed limit in river; water-skiing prohibited
Facilities:	parking for car and trailer (c), toilets at pub
Dues:	none
Charge:	approx. £5
Directions:	from Falmouth follow minor roads to Mawnan Smith then signs for Helford Passage: site is in front of 'Ferry Boat Inn'
Waters accessed:	Helford River and Falmouth Bay

Falmouth - Grove Place Boat Park and Slipway

Tel: (01326) 312285 (Harbour Office, 44 Arwenack Street)

Type:	large concrete ramp
Suits:	all craft except pwc and windsurfers
Availability:	all states of tide but 0900-1600 only in winter
Restrictions:	8 knot speed limit in Inner Harbour: water-skiing permitted in designated areas in Falmouth Bay; pwc and windsurfers prohibited
Facilities:	fuel from Yacht Haven, car parking nearby (c), trailers can be left on site (c), chandlery, diving supplies and outboard repairs all available in town; boats can be stored ashore (c), watersports centre adjacent with toilets, showers etc.
Dues:	included in launching fee
Charge:	approx. £5 daily, (£25 weekly and £75 annually)
Directions:	follow A39 to town centre: site is off main street
Waters accessed:	Fal Estuary and Falmouth Bay

Falmouth - Port Falmouth Boatyard, North Parade

Tel: (01326) 313248

Type:	concrete slipway (1:8)
Suits:	all craft except pwc
Availability:	approx. 3-4 hours either side HW 0800-1800
Restrictions:	8 knot speed limit in Inner Harbour: water-skiing permitted in designated areas in Falmouth Bay; pwc prohibited
Facilities:	diesel on site, petrol nearby, parking for car and trailer, toilets, and chandlery all on site, diving supplies and outboard repairs nearby; crane and other boatyard facilities on request
Dues:	none
Charge:	approx. £10 inc. car and trailer parking
Directions:	from Truro follow A39 to Penryn: site is on North Parade just before marina
Waters accessed:	Fal Estuary, Penryn River and Falmouth Bay

Penryn (Penryn River) - Church Slip

Tel: (01326) 373352 (Harbour Office, Penryn)

Type:	concrete and wooden slipway
Suits:	dinghies only
Availability:	approx. 2 hours either side HW by prior arrangement
Restrictions:	8 knot speed limit in Penryn river: pwc prohibited; narrow access roads
Facilities:	fuel nearby, parking for car only nearby, toilets, chandlery, diving supplies and outboard repairs all available nearby
Dues:	none
Charge:	none
Directions:	from Truro follow A39 to Falmouth: Penryn is at head of Penryn River and site is just below church off the Flushing road
Waters accessed:	Penryn River, Fal Estuary and Falmouth Bay

Flushing (Penryn River) - Quayside

Tel: (01326) 373352 (Harbour Office, Penryn)

Type:	concrete slipway
Suits:	dinghies only
Availability:	approx. 2 hours either side HW
Restrictions:	8 knot speed limit in Penryn River: pwc prohibited; limited access
Facilities:	fuel in village, parking for car and trailer on quay (c), pub
Dues:	none
Charge:	none
Directions:	from Truro follow A39 to Falmouth, turning off to Flushing in Penryn: site is opposite 'Seven Stars' pub
Waters accessed:	Penryn River, Fal Estuary and Falmouth Bay

Mylor (Mylor Creek) - Mylor Yacht Harbour
Tel: (01326) 372121

Type:	shallow concrete ramp
Suits:	all craft except pwc
Availability:	approx. 4 hours either side HW
Restrictions:	5 knot speed limit in Mylor Creek, water-skiing permitted in designated areas but pwc prohibited
Facilities:	fuel, parking for car and trailer (c), toilets and showers, chandlery, travel hoist, moorings, crane and restaurant all on site
Dues:	none
Charge:	approx. £3
Directions:	from Truro follow A39 to Falmouth, then brown signs to 'Yacht Harbour': slipway is next to restaurant
Waters accessed:	Mylor Creek, Fal Estuary and Falmouth Bay

Feock (Fal Estuary) - Loe Beach Boat Park
Tel: (01872) 864295 (Watersports Centre))

Type:	concrete ramp onto shingle foreshore
Suits:	all craft up to approx. 25'/7.6m LOA except pwc
Availability:	all states of tide
Restrictions:	8 knot speed limit north of Turnaware Bar: water-skiing permitted in designated areas but pwc prohibited; narrow access road
Facilities:	fuel from local garage, parking for car and trailer on site, toilets and cafe: all other facilities available in Falmouth or at marinas
Dues:	none
Charge:	approx. £3
Directions:	from Truro take the road to Feock and then follow signs to 'Loe Beach'
Waters accessed:	Fal Estuary and Falmouth Bay

Truro (Truro River) - Boscawen Park
Tel: (01872) 272130 (Harbour Master, Truro)

Type:	medium concrete ramp
Suits:	all craft
Availability:	approx. 3 hours either side HW
Restrictions:	8 knot speed limit in river: water-skiing permitted in designated areas in estuary and bay
Facilities:	fuel nearby, parking for car and trailer on site, toilets nearby: all other facilities available in Truro or Falmouth
Dues:	none
Charge:	none: (charge for boats over 20'/6.1m LOA)
Directions:	follow signs from Truro centre
Waters accessed:	Truro River, Fal Estuary and Falmouth Bay

Truro (Truro River) - Malpas Road, Sunny Corner
Tel: (01872) 272130 (Harbour Master)

Type:	steep right-angled concrete slipway onto muddy beach
Suits:	small powered craft, dinghies and small trailer-sailers
Availability:	approx. 2 hours either side HW by prior arrangement
Restrictions:	8 knot speed limit in river: water-skiing permitted in designated areas in estuary and bay
Facilities:	fuel nearby, limited parking for car only nearby, toilets, chandlery and other facilities in Truro or Falmouth
Dues:	none
Charge:	none
Directions:	turn left off A39 Truro by-pass at roundabout following signs to Malpas
Waters accessed:	Truro River, Fal Estuary and Falmouth Bay

St Just-in-Roseland (St Just Creek) - Pasco's Boatyard
Tel: (01326) 270269

Type:	shallow concrete ramp onto shingle foreshore
Suits:	all craft up to 20'/6.1m LOA
Availability:	all states of tide during daylight hours by prior arrangement
Restrictions:	5 knot speed limit in creek; water-skiing permitted in designated area; pwc and windsurfers prohibited; site can be busy in season and is exposed in strong SW winds
Facilities:	diesel, petrol nearby, parking for car nearby (c), trailer can be left on site, toilets, chandlery and outboard repairs all nearby
Dues:	none
Charge:	£3.50
Directions:	from Truro follow A3078 towards St Mawes: in St Just Lane, turn right into narrow road signposted 'St Just Church and Bar 1 mile'
Waters accessed:	St Just Creek, Fal Estuary and Falmouth Bay

St Mawes (Percuil River) - Harbour Slipway
Tel: (01326) 270553 (Harbour Master)

Type:	steep concrete ramp onto shingle foreshore
Suits:	all craft up to 25'/7.6m LOA except pwc
Availability:	approx. 3 hours either side HW (less at neaps) for direct launch but can be used longer if craft manhandled over beach; site available 0900-1800
Restrictions:	5 knot speed limit in harbour and river: water-skiing and pwc prohibited; access to site is through narrow and very congested streets; slipway is steep with 90° turn at bottom if launching over beach; there are locked posts at slipway head so Hbr Mr must be contacted prior to launching
Facilities:	fuel from garage (1mile), limited parking for car (c) in car park nearby (often full); visitor's moorings in river are available from the sailing club Tel: (01326) 270686

Dues:	included in launch fee
Charge:	approx. £6
Directions:	from St Austell follow A390 west taking the B3287 signposted 'Roseland Peninsula' then right onto A3078 to St Mawes: harbour is in centre of town
Waters accessed	Percuil River, Fal Estuary and Falmouth Bay

St Mawes (Percuil River) - Stoneworks Quay (St Mawes Sailing Club)
Tel (01326) 270686 or (01326) 270332/270528 (Quay Secretary/Manager)

Type:	concrete slipway onto soft mud
Suits:	dinghies and small powered craft up to 16'/4.9m LOA
Availability:	all states of tide by prior arrangement but very muddy at LW
Restrictions:	5 knot speed limit in harbour and river: site is private and permission to use must be obtained in advance: access is via a narrow lane with tight corners and there is a locked barrier with instructions for obtaining key displayed on quay notice board
Facilities:	parking for car and trailer nearby (c), toilets, temporary membership of club welcomed allowing access to all facilities during opening hours (all year 1000-1430 and additionally in season 1800-2300); moorings in Percuil River available (£6/night)
Dues:	none
Charge:	approx. £4 (£0.50 for tenders), payable to club
Directions:	from St Austell follow A390 west taking the B3287 signposted 'Roseland Peninsula' then right onto A3078 to St Mawes: access to site is down lane signed off Polvarth road approx ½ mile after petrol station
Waters accessed:	Percuil River, Fal Estuary and Falmouth Bay

St Mawes - Polvarth Boatyard (St Mawes Yacht Services)
Tel: (01326) 270475

Type:	shallow concrete ramp onto shingle foreshore
Suits:	all craft up to 20'/6.1m LOA
Availability:	approx. 4 hours either side HW during working hours by prior arrangment
Restrictions:	5 knot speed limit in Percuil River: access to site is via a steep and narrow lane with a locked barrier at top of slipway
Facilities:	fuel, parking for car and trailer (c), toilets, chandlery all available nearby
Dues:	none
Charge:	approx. £12
Directions:	from St Austell follow A390 west, taking the B3287 signposted 'Roseland Peninsula' then right onto A3078 to St Mawes: site is at end of Polvarth Lane and upstream of Polvarth Pt
Waters accessed:	Percuil River, Fal Estuary and Falmouth Bay

Percuil (Percuil River)- Percuil Boatyard Slipway
Tel: (01872) 580564

Type:	steep concrete slipway onto shingle beach
Suits:	dinghies and powerboats only
Availability:	most states of tide
Restrictions:	5 knot speed limit in Percuil River
Facilities:	parking for car and trailer, toilets, all yard facilities
Dues:	none
Charge:	none, but donation to RNLI box appreciated
Directions:	from St Austell follow A390 west, taking the B3287 signposted 'Roseland Peninsula' turning right onto A3078 to Trewithian and then following minor roads ; site is on east bank of river
Waters accessed:	Percuil River, Fal Estuary and Falmouth Bay

Place (Percuil River) - Place Manor

Type:	concrete slipway
Suits:	dinghies only
Availability:	approx. 4 hours either side HW
Restrictions:	5 knot speed limit in Percuil River
Facilities:	parking for car and trailer, boat park
Dues:	none
Charge:	none
Directions:	from St Austell follow A390 west, taking the B3287 signposted 'Roseland Peninsula' turning right onto A3078 to Trewithian and then following minor roads to Gerrans and signs to 'Place'
Waters accessed:	Percuil River, Fal Estuary and Falmouth Bay

Portscatho - Harbour Slip
Tel: (01872) 580616 (Harbour Master)

Type:	steep concrete and stone slipway onto sand
Suits:	shallow-draught craft up to 17'/5.2m LOA
Availability:	most states of tide by arrangement with Harbour Master
Restrictions:	5 mph speed limit in harbour and near beach: water-skiing and pwc permitted in designated areas offshore
Facilities:	fuel, parking for car and trailer, toilets, chandlery, diving supplies and outboard repairs all available nearby
Dues:	approx. £2.85
Charge:	no additional fee
Directions:	from St Austell follow A390 west, taking the B3287 signposted 'Roseland Peninsula' turning right onto A3078 to Trewithian and then follow minor roads to Portscatho
Waters accessed:	Gerrans Bay

Pentewan - Pentewan Sands Beach

Tel: (01726) 843485

Type:	short concrete ramp onto sandy beach
Suits:	all light craft except pwc
Availability:	all states of tide 1000-2000 from Whitsun to 14th Sept
Restrictions:	pwc are prohibited: no motor vehicles permitted on beach; beach is unsafe in onshore (east) winds; use by prior arrangement for park residents or season ticket holders only; all powered craft must have evidence of 3rd party insurance and are subject to site regulations; no dogs on park or beach
Facilities:	fuel nearby, parking for car and trailer, toilets, dinghy and canoe hire, caravan site all on site; diving supplies and outboard repairs available nearby
Dues:	yes
Charge:	approx. £7 per day (£30 per week) including parking
Directions:	from St Austell follow B3273 south towards Mevagissey: site is on right after approx. 4 miles
Waters accessed:	St Austell Bay

St Austell - Porthpean Beach

Tel: (01726) 223440 or Beach Office (in season) (01726) 76641

Type:	very steep concrete slipway onto soft sandy beach
Suits:	dinghies and small powered craft up to 10hp: no pwc
Availability:	all states of tide
Restrictions:	5 mph speed limit close to beach: pwc and water-skiing prohibited; 0900-1800 Easter to mid Sept, launching prohibited for craft over 10hp; part of beach buoyed off for bathing only in summer; launching area heavily used by Porthpean S.C.; vehicles can only be used on beach for launching and retrieval purposes and beach is only suitable for 4-wheel drive off-road vehicles
Facilities:	parking for car and trailer nearby (c), toilets, Porthpean S.C. at top of slip; beach attendants on duty Easter-mid Sept
Dues:	none
Charge:	none
Directions:	from A 390 St Austell by-pass approx. 300m east of 'Asda' roundabout, turn left onto minor road signposted 'Porthpean', then take 1st left after hospital to Porthpean Beach
Waters accessed:	St Austell Bay

Polkerris - Beach

Tel: (01726) 815142

Type:	concrete ramp
Suits:	all craft up to 18'/5.5m LOA
Availability:	all states of tide

Restrictions:	speed limit in harbour: water-skiing allowed offshore but no beach starts; no launching of power craft of 30hp and over on daily basis but moorings can be arranged for any powerboats; harbour exposed in SW gales; narrow access road
Facilities:	fuel nearby (1 mile), parking for car nearby (c) and trailer on site, toilets, pub and cafe; chandlery and other facilities in Fowey (3 miles)
Dues:	none
Charge:	approx. £2 includes trailer parking
Directions:	from St Austell follow A390 east turning right in Par onto A3082 towards Fowey: site is down minor road to left signposted 'Polkerris and Beach'
Waters accessed:	St Austell Bay

Fowey (Fowey Harbour) - Caffa Mill Car/Dinghy Park

Tel: (01726) 832471/2 (Harbour Office, Albert Quay)

Type:	concrete slipway onto shingle
Suits:	craft up to 25'/7.6m LOA: no windsurfers or pwc
Availability:	all states of tide
Restrictions:	6 knot speed limit in harbour: water-skiing, windsurfers and pwc prohibited in harbour; access to site is via narrow roads
Facilities:	fuel nearby, parking for car and trailer on site for limited time (c), toilets on site, other facilities in town
Dues:	on application to Harbour Office
Charge:	approx. £1
Directions:	follow signs from roundabout by 'Four Turnings' service station to 'Fowey Jetties' or 'Bodinnick car ferry': these will lead to the Caffa Mill car park on the Fowey side of the river
Waters accessed:	Fowey Harbour

Mixtow Pill (Fowey Harbour) - Slipway

Tel: (01726) 832471/2 (Harbour Office, Albert Quay)

Type:	concrete slipway approx. 8'/2.4m wide
Suits:	dinghies and very small powered craft: no windsurfers or pwc
Availability:	approx. 1½ hours either side HW
Restrictions:	6 knot speed limit in harbour: water-skiing, windsurfers and pwc prohibited in harbour; access is via narrow one-way roads with sharp bends
Facilities:	diesel nearby, no parking; other facilities in Fowey
Dues:	on application to Harbour Office
Charge:	none
Directions:	turn off at Lostwithiel following signs to Lerryn, then St Veep and Mixtow
Waters accessed:	Fowey Harbour

Bodinnick (Fowey Harbour) - Yeate Farm Slipway
Tel: (01726) 870256 (D.J. and A.M. Oliver)

Type:	steep concrete slipway (1:6) onto hard beach, then mud
Suits:	all craft except pwc
Availability:	approx. 5 hours either side HW from 0900 to dusk
Restrictions:	6 knot speed limit in river: water-skiing, windsurfing and pwc prohibited: access is via steep narrow road and through security gate
Facilities:	fuel (5 miles), parking for car and trailer on site (c), toilets nearby, chandlery and diving supplies (1 mile), outboard repairs (3 miles); small caravan site on farm, cottage to let, boats can be stored and tractor and hoist available up to 4 tonnes
Dues:	on application to Harbour Office Tel:(01726) 832471/2
Charge:	approx. £4
Directions:	from A38 Liskeard by-pass, fork left at Dobwalls onto the A390: turn left at East Taphouse onto the B3359 and follow signs to the 'Bodinnick Ferry'; farm is 1/2 mile east of ferry
Waters accessed:	Fowey Harbour

Polruan (Fowey Harbour) - Polruan Quay Slip
Tel: (01726) 832471/2 (Harbour Office, Albert Quay)

Type:	wide concrete slipway onto beach
Suits:	dinghies and small powered craft only: no windsurfers or pwc
Availability:	approx. 3 hours either side HW
Restrictions:	6 knot speed limit in harbour: water-skiing, windsurfers and pwc prohibited; narrow access roads; area may be very congested
Facilities:	fuel on quay, no parking, toilets and chandlery in village
Dues:	on application to Harbour Office
Charge:	yes
Directions:	from Lostwithiel follow minor roads to Polruan
Waters accessed:	Fowey Harbour

West Looe - Millpool Boatyard (Norman Pearn & Co Ltd)
Tel: (01503) 262244

Type:	concrete slipway
Suits:	all craft
Availability:	approx. 4 hours either side HW
Restrictions:	5 knot speed limit in harbour and for some distance offshore: water-skiing allowed in open sea; site is above bridge so is not suitable for boats with masts
Facilities:	fuel from petrol station on opposite side of river, parking for car and trailer on site (c), toilets nearby, chandlery, outboard repairs and all yard facilities available on site, diving supplies nearby
Dues:	none

Charge:	approx. £4
Directions:	from Plymouth take the A38 then A387 following signs to Looe: cross over bridge into West Looe taking the second turning right, going down hill to mini round-about then heading back towards Looe
Waters accessed:	Looe River and Bay

West Looe - The Quay

Tel: (01503) 262839 (Harbour Office)

Type:	concrete slipway
Suits:	all craft
Availability:	approx. 2½ hours either side HW by prior arrangement
Restrictions:	5 knot speed limit in harbour and for some distance offshore: water-skiing allowed in open sea
Facilities:	fuel nearby, parking for car nearby (c), trailers can be left in Millpool car park (c), toilets and shower, chandlery, outboard repairs, diving supplies, moorings all nearby
Dues:	none
Charge:	approx. £6: weekly/monthly rates available
Directions:	from Plymouth take the A38 then A387 following signs to Looe: cross over bridge into W. Looe taking left turn to Quay
Waters accessed:	Looe Harbour and Bay

Millendreath - Millendreath Holiday Village

Tel: (01503) 263281

Type:	launching by hand or tractor launching
Suits:	all craft except pwc
Availability:	all states of tide 0830-1800
Restrictions:	5 knot speed limit within 300m of beach: no vehicles allowed near slipway
Facilities:	parking for car and trailer (c), toilets, cafe, shop, pub and clubhouse all on site: fuel, chandlery and outboard repairs in Looe
Dues:	none
Charge:	approx. £30
Directions:	from Plymouth take the A38 then A387 following signs to Looe, turn left onto B3253 at Shorta Cross and follow signs
Waters accessed:	Looe Bay

Downderry - Downderry Slipway

Tel: (01579) 341343 (Water Safety Officer, Caradon District Council)

Type:	shallow concrete ramp onto shingle foreshore
Suits:	sailing dinghies, small powered craft and speedboats: no pwc
Availability:	approx. 2 hours either side HW for direct launching but craft can be manhandled over the beach at all states of tide

Restrictions:	narrow access to site: there is a voluntary code of conduct inshore; pwc prohibited
Facilities:	parking for car and trailer, toilets, shop and pub nearby
Dues:	none
Charge:	none
Directions:	from Plymouth follow the A38, A374, A387 and B3247 then signs from village: site is 3 miles east of Looe
Waters accessed:	Whitsand Bay

Portwrinkle - Harbour Slip

Tel: (01579) 341343 (Water Safety Officer, Caradon District Council)

Type:	steep concrete ramp onto shingle foreshore
Suits:	sailing dinghies and small powered craft: no pwc
Availability:	at all states of tide or near HW for a direct launch
Restrictions:	narrow access may be obstructed by lockable bollards - key is with Harbour Master (see notice on site): there is a voluntary code of conduct inshore; pwc and water-skiing prohibited
Facilities:	parking for car and trailer (c), toilets and hotel nearby
Dues:	none
Charge:	none
Directions:	from Plymouth follow the A38/A374, then turn right onto B3247
Waters accessed:	Whitsand Bay

Cawsand (Plymouth Harbour) - Cawsand Bay Slip

Tel: (01579) 341343 (Water Safety Officer, Caradon District Council)

Type:	short concrete ramp onto pebble beach
Suits:	small trailed craft: no windsurfers
Availability:	approx. 3 hours either side HW
Restrictions:	10 knot speed limit in harbour with designated high speed areas: access to site is via a narrow passage (max. 7'/2.1m wide); no trailers or vehicles to be left on slipway or beach; windsurfing prohibited
Facilities:	parking for car and trailer nearby (c), limited boat parking, toilets
Dues:	none
Charge:	none
Directions:	follow B3247 towards Kingsand and down to public car park or directly to water front via 'The Bound' just off St Andrew Place and next to the Cawsand Bay Hotel
Waters accessed:	Cawsand Bay, Plymouth Sound and the English Channel

Millbrook (Plymouth Harbour) - Flood Prevention Slipway
Tel: (01579) 341343 (Water Safety Officer, Caradon District Council)

Type:	concrete ramp with timber edge 20'/6.1m wide with sharp drop at end
Suits:	all craft up to 20'/6.1m LOA
Availability:	approx. 1 hour either side HW
Restrictions:	10 knot speed limit in harbour with designated high speed areas: vehicle access to south side only
Facilities:	limited parking for car and trailer on roadside
Dues:	none
Charge:	none
Directions:	follow B3247 east towards Millbrook, turning left to Anderton : slip is situated on left-hand side
Waters accessed:	Millbrook Lake, Hamoaze and Plymouth Sound

Millbrook (Plymouth Harbour) - Southdown Marina, Southdown Quay
Tel: (01752) 823084

Type:	launching over shingle hard
Suits:	all craft including sailboards and pwc
Availability:	approx. 2 hours either side HW by prior arrangement
Restrictions:	10 knot speed limit in harbour with designated high speed areas: slipway must be booked in advance
Facilities:	diesel on site, petrol nearby, parking for car and trailer, toilets
Dues:	included in launching fee
Charge:	approx. £10
Directions:	from Plymouth take the A374 via the Torpoint ferry then the B3247 to Millbrook, or go along the A38 to Trerucefoot roundabout, taking the A374 onto the B3247 and turning off to Millbrook
Waters accessed:	River Tamar, Plymouth Harbour and Sound

Torpoint (Plymouth Harbour) - Public Slip, Marine Drive
Tel: (01579) 341343 (Water Safety Officer, Caradon District Council)

Type:	concrete ramp onto pebble beach
Suits:	small craft
Availability:	approx. 2 hours either side HW
Restrictions:	10 knot speed limit in harbour with designated high speed areas: no parking on slipway
Facilities:	limited parking for car and trailer opposite site
Dues:	none
Charge:	none
Directions:	turn right off A374 Antony Road into Marine Drive: site is at the turning and access is narrow
Waters accessed:	River Tamar, Plymouth Harbour and Sound

Torpoint (Plymouth Harbour) - Torpoint Yacht Harbour Ltd
Tel: (01752) 813658

Type:	shingle hard
Suits:	dinghies and small powered craft
Availability:	approx. 5 hours either side HW
Restrictions:	10 knot speed limit in harbour with designated high speed areas
Facilities:	diesel on site, petrol from garage, parking for car and trailer and chandlery on site
Dues:	none
Charge:	none
Directions:	from Plymouth follow A374 via Torpoint Ferry and then signs to 'Ballast Quay'
Waters accessed:	River Tamar, Plymouth Harbour and Sound

Torpoint (Plymouth Harbour) - Wilcove
Tel: (01579) 341343 (Water Safety Officer, Caradon County Council)

Type:	launching from road over muddy foreshore
Suits:	small craft
Availability:	at HW only
Restrictions:	10 knot speed limit in harbour with designated high speed areas
Facilities:	limited parking in street, pub nearby
Dues:	none
Charge:	none
Directions:	following A374 to Torpoint, turn left after Maryfield to Wilcove waterfront via Pengelly Lane
Waters accessed:	River Tamar, Plymouth Harbour and Sound

Landrake (River Lynher) - Boating World
Tel: (01752) 851679

Type:	steep concrete ramp
Suits:	all craft up to 36'/11m LOA
Availability:	approx. 3 hours either side HW by prior arrangement
Restrictions:	5 knot speed limit in river: water-skiing, pwc and wind-surfers prohibited; access restricted to 14'/4.3m height and 11'/3.4m width
Facilities:	diesel, parking for car and trailer, toilets, chandlery, boat repairs, outboard repairs, storage, cafe all on site
Dues:	none
Charge:	approx. £8
Directions:	from Plymouth follow A38 west to Landrake turning left when signposted 'Boating World' and following signs for 2 miles, turning left by pub in village
Waters accessed:	Rivers Lynher, Tamar and St Germans and Plymouth Harbour

Saltash (River Tamar) - Old Ferry Slip, Old Ferry Road

Tel: (01579) 341343 (Water Safety Officer, Caradon District Council)

Type:	concrete slipway on north side of Pier
Suits:	small craft
Availability:	approx. 3 hours either side HW
Restrictions:	10 knot speed limit in harbour with designated high speed areas
Facilities:	fuel, parking for car and trailer, toilets and pubs all nearby
Dues:	none
Charge:	none
Directions:	turn off the B3271 North Road east-bound onto Old Ferry Road and continue under bridges: site is on downstream side of Royal Albert Bridge and on north side of pier
Waters accessed:	River Tamar, Plymouth Harbour and Sound

Saltash (River Tamar) - Brunel Green Slipway

Tel: (01579) 341343 (Water Safety Officer, Caradon District Council)

Type:	concrete slipway
Suits:	small craft
Availability:	approx. 2 hours either side HW for direct launch
Restrictions:	10 knot speed limit in harbour with designated high speed areas: narrow access to site
Facilities:	fuel, parking for car and trailer, dinghy park, toilets, pubs and club all nearby
Dues:	none
Charge:	none
Directions:	from B3271 North Road, east-bound, turn left onto Old Ferry Road: site is between Brunel Green and Jubilee car park
Waters accessed:	River Tamar, Hamoaze and Plymouth Sound

Cargreen (River Tamar) - Old Ferry Slip, next Crooked Spaniards Inn

Tel: (01752) 842830 (Crooked Spaniards Inn)

Type:	concrete slipway
Suits:	sailing dinghies and small powered craft
Availability:	at all states of tide except LWS
Restrictions:	10 knot speed limit in harbour with designated high speed areas: narrow and steep access road into private car park
Facilities:	parking for car and trailer on site (c), toilets in pub, pub and shops, overnight moorings
Dues:	none
Charge:	none
Directions:	turn off A388 Saltash to Callington road following signs to Cargreen: site is in village and adjacent to the Crooked Spaniards Inn
Waters accessed:	River Tamar, Hamoaze and Plymouth Sound

Calstock (River Tamar) - Riverside

Tel: (01579) 341343 (Water Safety Officer, Caradon District Council)

Type:	steep concrete slipway; min. width 10'/3m
Suits:	craft up to 20'/6.1m LOA
Availability:	approx. 1 hour either side HW
Restrictions:	10 knot speed limit in harbour with designated high speed areas; access to site is narrow and steep
Facilities:	parking (often congested) for car and trailer on site (c), toilets, pubs and shops
Dues:	none
Charge:	none
Directions:	follow signs from the A390 Liskeard to Tavistock road, turning right after St Ann's Chapel and following road to river
Waters accessed:	upper navigable reaches of River Tamar and Plymouth Sound

Calstock (River Tamar) - Calstock Steam Packet & River Nav.Co.Ltd.

Tel: (01822) 833331

Type:	medium concrete slipway
Suits:	all craft except windsurfers and pwc
Availability:	approx. 3 hours either side HW
Restrictions:	10 knot speed limit in harbour with designated high speed areas; larger craft only by prior arrangement to ensure clear access
Facilities:	diesel on site, limited parking for car and trailer, toilets & showers, limited chandlery, outboard repairs, moorings, winter storage, boat lift and all yard facilities on site; pub & shops nearby
Dues:	none
Charge:	£25 per season
Directions:	follow signs from the A390 Tavistock to Callington road
Waters accessed:	upper navigable reaches of River Tamar and Plymouth Sound

Bere Alston (River Tavy) - Weir Quay Boatyard, Herons' Reach

Tel: (01822) 840474

Type:	concrete slipway
Suits:	all craft: facilities for launching boats up to 12 tons
Availability:	all states of tide by prior arrangement
Restrictions:	10 knot speed limit in harbour with designated high speed areas: phone in advance to advise arrival and requirements
Facilities:	diesel on site, petrol nearby, parking for car and trailer on site , toilets and showers, chandlery, storage ashore, moorings and all yard facilities on site
Dues:	none
Charge:	approx. £12; crane, £10.50 per m
Directions:	from Tavistock, take the A390 Liskeard road, turning left at the Harvest Home pub for Bere Alston: once in the village, take the lane to Weir Quay, turning left at the river
Waters accessed:	Rivers Tavy and Tamar, Plymouth Harbour and Sound

Bere Alston (River Tavy) - Weir Quay Slipway
Tel: (01822) 615911 (West Devon Borough Council)

Type:	wide coarse gravel slipway
Suits:	small craft
Availability:	approx. 3 hours either side HW
Restrictions:	10 knot speed limit in harbour with designated high speed areas
Facilities:	fuel nearby, parking for car and trailer on site, boat-yard and sailing club nearby
Dues:	none
Charge:	none
Directions:	from Tavistock, take the A390 Liskeard road, turning left at the Harvest Home pub for Bere Alston: once in the village, take the lane to Weir Quay, turning left at the river: site is beyond Weir Quay sailing club
Waters accessed:	Rivers Tavy and Tamar, Plymouth Harbour and Sound

Plymouth (River Tamar) - Saltash Passage Slipway, Wolesey Road
Tel: (01752) 224304 (Harbour Master, Plymouth City Council)

Type:	stepped granite slipway
Suits:	small craft
Availability:	approx. 3 hours either side HW
Restrictions:	10 knot speed limit in harbour with designated high speed areas: sharp 90° turn from narrow road
Facilities:	fuel nearby, limited parking for car and trailer on site, toilets opposite, dinghy park on site
Dues:	none
Charge:	none
Directions:	from the A38 on the east side of the Tamar Bridge, turn left into Pembros Road, then right down Normandy Hill following Wolesey Road onto the water front
Waters accessed:	River Tamar and Plymouth Harbour and Sound

Plymouth (River Tamar)- Ferry House Inn Slipway
Tel: (01752) 224304 (Harbour Master, Plymouth City Council)

Type:	wide moderate/steep concrete slipway
Suits:	small craft
Availability:	approx. 3 hours either side HW
Restrictions:	10 knot speed limit in harbour with designated high speed areas; slipway surface is poor
Facilities:	fuel nearby, limited roadside parking, toilets nearby
Dues:	none
Charge:	none
Directions:	from the A38 on the east side of the Tamar Bridge, turn left into Pembros Road and right down Normandy Hill following Wolesey Road along waterfront for approx. 200m
Waters accessed:	River Tamar and Plymouth Harbour and Sound

Plymouth (River Tamar) - Pottery Quay Slipway, Tamar Canal
Tel: (01752) 224304 (Harbour Master, Plymouth City Council)

Type:	gentle concrete slipway
Suits:	small craft
Availability:	approx. 1 hour either side HW
Restrictions:	10 knot speed limit in harbour with designated high speed areas; gates to slipway
Facilities:	fuel nearby, limited roadside parking for car and trailer
Dues:	none
Charge:	none
Directions:	follow A 374 west from Plymouth city centre towards Torpoint ferry: on Pottery Road turn left into John St. and follow road to water's edge
Waters accessed:	Tamar Canal, River Tamar and Plymouth Harbour and Sound

Plymouth (River Tamar) - North Corner Slipway, Cornwall Street
Tel: (01752) 224304 (Harbour Master, Plymouth City Council)

Type:	gentle concrete slipway
Suits:	small craft without masts
Availability:	approx. 3 hour either side HW
Restrictions:	10 knot speed limit in harbour with designated high speed areas: there is a 12'/3.6m height restriction
Facilities:	fuel nearby, limited street parking
Dues:	none
Charge:	none
Directions:	follow A 374 west from Plymouth city centre towards Torpoint ferry: turn left immediately after RN Dockyard along Granby Way, Albany Street and to the end of Cornwall St
Waters accessed:	River Tamar and Plymouth Harbour and Sound

Plymouth (River Tamar) - Mutton Cove Slipway
Tel: (01752) 224304 (Harbour Master, Plymouth City Council)

Type:	steep narrow granite cobbled slipway
Suits:	small craft
Availability:	approx. 3 hours either side HW
Restrictions:	10 knot speed limit in harbour with designated high speed areas; narrow access to slipway
Facilities:	fuel nearby, parking within harbour walls for 10 cars, toilets on site, all other facilities at Mayflower Marina
Dues:	none
Charge:	none
Directions:	follow A374 west past Cumberland Centre and turn left down Mount St adjoining James St, to waterfront
Waters accessed:	River Tamar and Plymouth Harbour and Sound

Plymouth - 'Commando Beach', Richmond Walk

Tel: (01752) 224304 (Harbour Master, Plymouth City Council)

Type:	wide and gentle concrete slipway
Suits:	all craft
Availability:	all times except LWS
Restrictions:	10 knot speed limit in harbour with designated high speed areas; access road narrow and sometimes congested
Facilities:	fuel from marina adjacent, parking for car and trailer on site or at marina (c), toilets on site (April-Sept), all other facilities at marina
Dues:	none
Charge:	none
Directions:	head through Plymouth city centre, down Union St and straight over at Stonehouse roundabout (in the direction of the Torpoint ferry) taking the first left into Richmond Walk: site is adjacent the Mayflower Marina
Waters accessed:	River Tamar and Plymouth Harbour and Sound

Plymouth - Teats Hill Slipway

Tel: (01752) 224304 (Harbour Master, Plymouth City Council)

Type:	wide and gentle concrete slipway
Suits:	all craft
Availability:	approx. 3 hours either side HW
Restrictions:	10 knot speed limit in harbour with designated high speed areas
Facilities:	fuel nearby, very limited parking
Dues:	none
Charge:	none
Directions:	from A374 Exeter Street, turn right into Sutton Rd signed 'Coxside'; then right into Teats Hill Road and slipway is at end of road
Waters accessed:	River Tamar and Plymouth Harbour and Sound

Coxside (Plymouth Harbour) - Queen Anne's Battery Marina

Tel: (01752) 671142

Type:	wide shallow concrete slipway
Suits:	all craft up to 30'/9m LOA
Availability:	approx. 4½ hours either side HW
Restrictions:	4 knot speed limit in marina: 10 knot speed limit in harbour with designated high speed areas: locked barriers across access 2400 - 0600; all visitors must report to the marina office
Facilities:	fuel, parking for car and trailer(c), toilets & showers, chandlery, diving supplies, outboard repairs, sail repairs and many other facilities available at marina

Dues:	included in launching fee
Charge:	approx. £7
Directions:	from the A38, follow signs to the city centre and then to Coxside; from Sutton Rd turn right into Teats Hill Rd and entrance to marina is on left
Waters accessed:	Plymouth Sound and English Channel

Plymouth (Cattewater) - Oreston Slipway

Tel: (01752) 224304 (Harbour Master, Plymouth City Council)

Type:	two concrete slipways
Suits:	small craft
Availability:	approx. 3 hours either side HW
Restrictions:	10 knot speed limit in harbour with designated high speed areas
Facilities:	fuel nearby, off-street parking for car and trailer
Dues:	none
Charge:	none
Directions:	from the A379 go east over Laira Bridge, turning right at first roundabout and then follow Rollis Park Road to the quay
Waters accessed:	Cattewater, Plymouth Sound and English Channel

Plymouth (Cattewater) - Plymouth Yacht Haven, Shaw Way

Tel: (01752) 404231

Type:	wide shallow concrete ramp with drop at end
Suits:	all craft
Availability:	at all states of tide by prior arrangement
Restrictions:	8 knot speed limit in Cattewater: 4 knots in Sutton Channel and 10 knots in harbour with designated high speed areas
Facilities:	diesel on site, petrol nearby, parking for car and trailer on site (c), toilets & showers, chandlery, diving supplies, outboard repairs and all yard facilities available on site
Dues:	no additional charge
Charge:	approx. £2.35 per metre
Directions:	from A 38, follow signs to Plymouth city centre along A374, Embankment Rd staying in right-hand lane. After approx. 1 mile follow signs for Kingsbridge (A379) which takes you across Laira Bridge. At 1st roundabout turn right to Plymstock and follow road to Hooe past McMullins Garage on left then going up hill; continue along this road to Mount Batten
Waters accessed:	Hooe Lake, Cattewater and Plymouth Sound

Plymouth (Cattewater) - Mount Batten Slip

Tel: (01752) 224304 (Harbour Master, Plymouth City Council)

Type:	wide gentle concrete and stone slip
Suits:	all craft
Availability:	all times except LWS
Restrictions:	10 knot speed limit in harbour with designated high speed areas

Facilities:	fuel from marina adjacent, parking for car and trailer nearby, all other facilities at marina
Dues:	none
Charge:	none
Directions:	from A 38, follow signs to Plymouth city centre along A374, Embankment Rd staying in right-hand lane. After approx. 1 mile follow signs for Kingsbridge (A379) which takes you across Laira Bridge. At 1st roundabout turn right to Plymstock and follow road to Hooe past McMullins Garage on left then going up hill; continue along this road to Mount Batten; site is south of jetty
Waters accessed:	Hooe Lake, Cattewater and Plymouth Sound

Plymouth - Fort Bovisand Slipway

Tel: (01803) 861141 (South Hams District Council))

Type:	concrete slipway
Suits:	all craft
Availability:	at all states of tide
Restrictions:	10 knot speed limit in harbour with designated high speed areas
Facilities:	limited parking and toilets on site
Dues:	none
Charge:	approx. £6
Directions:	follow A379 east towards Plymstock, then signs south to Bovisand Beach via Staddon Fort and continue along rough track to Bovisand Pier
Waters accessed:	Plymouth Sound

Newton Ferrers (River Yealm) - Bridgend Quay, Noss Mayo

Tel: (01752) 872533 (Harbour Master)

Type:	shallow concrete ramp onto shingle and mud
Suits:	all craft up to 20'/6.1m LOA except pwc
Availability:	approx. 2½ hours either side HW by prior arrangement
Restrictions:	6 knot speed limit in harbour and estuary: water-skiing and pwc prohibited; access is via very narrow roads with tight corners
Facilities:	very limited parking for car and trailer (c), toilets nearby
Dues:	none (unless stay exceeds two weeks)
Charge:	approx. £15 per week; no daily charge
Directions:	from Kingsbridge follow A379 towards Plymouth, turning onto B3186: site is at head of creek
Waters accessed:	Newton Creek, River Yealm and Wembury Bay

Bantham (River Avon)

Tel: (01548) 561196 (Harbour Master)

Type:	steep stone track to foreshore: 4-wheel drive vehicle necessary
Suits:	dinghies and small powered craft
Availability:	approx. 2 hours either side HW

Restrictions:	8 knot speed limit in harbour: water-skiing permitted in designated area only; beware strong tidal currents in river entrance; access road is very narrow and slip can be blocked by parked cars
Facilities:	parking for car nearby (c), pub 'The Sloop' and toilets nearby
Dues:	none
Charge:	none
Directions:	from Kingsbridge follow A379 towards Plymouth and through Churchstow, turning off at Bantham roundabout
Waters accessed:	River Avon and Bigbury Bay

Hope Cove - Old Lifeboat Slip, Inner Hope

Tel: (01548) 560928 (Ray Staff)

Type:	shallow concrete ramp onto firm sand
Suits:	all craft
Availability:	all states of tide 0900-1800
Restrictions:	5 knot speed limit inshore of buoys: water-skiing permitted offshore; all craft are launched at the discretion of the Hbr Mr
Facilities:	parking for car and trailer (c) nearby and toilets on site; boats can be parked by arrangement; Harbour Master on duty Easter to Sept
Dues:	none
Charge:	approx. £4; £15 per week, £40 per year
Directions:	from A38 (Exeter-Plymouth road) take the A384 to Totnes then A381 to Malborough via Kingsbridge: turn right and follow minor roads to Hope Cove: site is old lifeboat slip at Inner Hope
Waters accessed:	Hope Cove and Bigbury Bay

Salcombe Harbour - South Sands

Tel: (01548) 843791 (Harbour Office, Whitestrand)

Type:	short shallow concrete slipway onto firm sand
Suits:	all craft up to 18'/5.5m LOA except pwc
Availability:	all states of tide
Restrictions:	8 knot speed limit: pwc and water-skiing prohibited in harbour; access is across beach so 4-wheel drive vehicle recommended; all craft must have 3rd party insurance cover
Facilities:	fuel from barge in harbour, parking for car and trailer (c) and toilets on site , moorings up to 20'/6.1m LOA, all other facilities in town
Dues:	approx. £1.10 per m (max. 3 days)
Charge:	no additional fee
Directions:	from A38 (Exeter-Plymouth road) take the A384 to Totnes then A381 to Salcombe via Kingsbridge: site is 1 mile south of town centre on south side of beach
Waters accessed:	Salcombe Harbour

Salcombe - Whitestrand Quay

Tel: (01548) 843791 (Harbour Office, Whitestrand)

Type:	medium concrete slipway onto shingle
Suits:	small powered craft and sailing dinghies: no pwc
Availability:	approx. 3 hours either side HW for direct launch or at all states of tide over shingle
Restrictions:	8 knot speed limit in harbour: pwc, diving and water-skiing prohibited; access is narrow and congested (Batson Park slipway is best)
Facilities:	fuel nearby, parking for car and trailer nearby (c), toilets on site, most other facilities available in town
Dues:	approx £1.10 per metre (max. 3 days)
Charge:	no separate fee
Directions:	from A38 (Exeter-Plymouth road) take the A384 to Totnes then A381 to Salcombe via Kingsbridge: site is in car park in centre of town adjacent to Harbour Office
Waters accessed:	Salcombe Harbour

Salcombe - Batson Creek Boat Park Slip

Tel: (01803) 861358 (Boat Park Attendant, 0900-1800)

Type:	large shallow concrete slipway onto shingle foreshore
Suits:	all craft except pwc
Availability:	all states of tide
Restrictions:	8 knot speed limit in harbour: water-skiing, pwc and diving prohibited in harbour
Facilities:	fuel nearby, parking for car, boat and trailer on site (c), toilets and other facilities nearby; 10 ton crane available from Winters Marine Tel: (01548) 843580 or Harbour Office Tel: (01548) 843791; advance bookings (advisable in summer) through Harbour Office
Dues:	approx. £1.10 per m (max. 3 days)
Charge:	no separate fee
Directions:	from A38 (Exeter-Plymouth road) take the A384 to Totnes then A381 to Salcombe via Kingsbridge: site is in Batson car park to north of town centre off Gould Road
Waters accessed:	Salcombe Harbour

Kingsbridge (Salcombe Harbour) - Squares Slip

Tel: (01548) 843791 (Harbour Office, Whitestrand, Salcombe)

Type:	shallow concrete slipway
Suits:	all craft except pwc
Availability:	approx. 2 hours either side HW or at HW for larger craft (up to 5'/1.5m draught)
Restrictions:	8 knot speed limit in harbour: water-skiing, pwc and diving prohibited; 15 ton weight limit and no parking on slipway
Facilities:	fuel nearby, parking for car and trailer on site (c), toilets and other facilities available nearby
Dues:	approx. £1.10 per m (max. 3 days)
Charge:	no separate fee

Directions: from A38 (Exeter-Plymouth road) take the A384 to Totnes then A381 to Kingsbridge: site is at Squares Quay at head of estuary

Waters accessed: Salcombe Harbour

Dartmouth (River Dart) - Higher Ferry Slip (South Side)

Tel: (01803) 832337 (Dart Harbour Authority)

Type:	concrete slipway
Suits:	all craft
Availability:	all states of tide
Restrictions:	6 knot speed limit in river: water-skiing prohibited
Facilities:	fuel from barge, parking for car and trailer (c) and toilets nearby: other facilties at marinas or in Dartmouth
Dues:	approx. £2.28
Charge:	no separate fee
Directions:	from A38 (Exeter-Plymouth road) take the A384 to Totnes: turn onto A381 and at Halwell take the A3122 following signs to ferry

Waters accessed: River Dart and Start Bay

Dartmouth - Dart Marina, Sandquay

Tel: (01803) 834582

Type:	2 concrete slipways
Suits:	all craft except pwc
Availability:	all states of tide
Restrictions:	6 knot speed limit in river: water-skiing, pwc, windsurfing and diving prohibited
Facilities:	diesel on site, petrol nearby, parking for car and trailer and toilets on site, chandlery and outboard repairs available nearby
Dues:	approx. £2.28
Charge:	approx. £36 + vat
Directions:	turn off A38 (Exeter-Plymouth road) onto A384 following signs to Totnes then onto A381 and at Halwell take the A3122 following signs to Higher Ferry: site is just north of ferry adjacent Hotel

Waters accessed: River Dart and Start Bay

Dittisham (River Dart) - Ham Car Park

Tel: (01803) 832337 (Dart Harbour Authority)

Type:	shingle foreshore
Suits:	small craft only
Availability:	near HW: launching difficult at neaps
Restrictions:	6 knot speed limit in river: water-skiing prohibited; access is via narrow congested roads and steep hill
Facilities:	parking for car and trailer on site (c), toilets
Dues:	approx. £2.28
Charge:	no separate fee

Directions:	from A38 take the A384 following signs to Totnes, turning onto A381 and at Halwell take the A3122 to Dartmouth: follow signs to Dittisham and access is through car park
Waters accessed:	River Dart and Start Bay

Totnes (River Dart) - Ashford Slip, Mill Tail (off The Plains)

Tel: (01803) 832337 (Dart Harbour Authority)

Type:	concrete slipway
Suits:	all craft
Availability:	approx. 3 hours either side HW
Restrictions:	6 knot speed limit in river: water-skiing prohibited
Facilities:	fuel, parking for car and trailer in public car park (c), toilets and chandlery all nearby
Dues:	approx. £2.28
Charge:	no separate fee
Directions:	from A38 take the A384 following signs to Totnes: site is on west bank, approx. 100m below road bridge and opposite Tourist Information Centre
Waters accessed:	River Dart and Start Bay

Totnes (River Dart) - Longmarsh (Steamer Quay)

Tel: (01803) 832337 (Dart Harbour Authority)

Type:	concrete slipway
Suits:	sailing dinghies and small powered craft
Availability:	approx. 2 hours either side HW
Restrictions:	6 knot speed limit in harbour: water-skiing prohibited
Facilities:	parking for car on site and for trailer nearby (c), toilets nearby
Dues:	approx. £2.28
Charge:	no separate fee
Directions:	from Exeter follow A38 turning off onto A384/A385: site is in town centre on east bank of river approx. 1/2 mile south of the town bridge
Waters accessed:	River Dart and Start Bay

Stoke Gabriel (River Dart)

Tel: (01803) 832337 (Dart Harbour Authority)

Type:	concrete slipway onto shingle
Suits:	sailing dinghies and small powered craft
Availability:	approx. 3 hours either side HWS, or 2 hours either side HWN
Restrictions:	6 knot speed limit in river: water-skiing prohibited; narrow access roads
Facilities:	fuel nearby, limited parking for car (c) but not trailer and toilets on site
Dues:	approx. £2.28
Charge:	no additional fee
Directions:	from Exeter follow A38 turning off onto A384/A385 to Totnes; turn right after town and follow signs to Stoke Gabriel
Waters accessed:	River Dart and Start Bay

Galmpton Creek (River Dart) - Dartside Quay

Tel: (01803) 845445

Type:	concrete slipway with locked barrier
Suits:	dinghies and small powered craft
Availability:	approx. 2-3 hours either side HW during working hours
Restrictions:	6 knot speed limit in river: water-skiing prohibited; cars with trailers only, no commercial vehicles through village
Facilities:	limited parking for car and trailer, toilets, chandlery, outboard repairs all on site, diving supplies nearby
Dues:	approx. £2.28
Charge:	approx. £11.75
Directions:	from Exeter follow A38 turning off onto A384/A385 to Totnes, then take A3022 towards Brixham and turn right in Galmpton village
Waters accessed:	River Dart and Start Bay

Greenway Quay (River Dart)

Tel: (01803) 844010

Type:	concrete slipway
Suits:	all craft
Availability:	approx. 4 hours either side HW
Restrictions:	6 knot speed limit in river: water-skiing prohibited; narrow access roads
Facilities:	parking for car and trailer on site (c)
Dues:	approx. £2.28
Charge:	approx. £5
Directions:	follow A3022 from Paignton, turning right at Galmpton: site is opposite Dittisham Ferry
Waters accessed:	River Dart and Start Bay

Kingswear (River Dart) - Slipway

Tel: (01803) 832337 (Dart Harbour Authority)

Type:	cobbled stone slipway
Suits:	dinghies and small powered craft up to 16'/4.9m LOA
Availability:	approx. 4 hours either side HW
Restrictions:	6 knot speed limit in river: water-skiing prohibited; access is via steep no-through road leading to Lower Ferry, often with queue of vehicles
Facilities:	fuel from barge in river, parking for car and trailer nearby (c), toilets, chandlery and outboard repairs all available in nearby marina
Dues:	approx. £2.28
Charge:	no separate charge
Directions:	from Exeter follow A38/A380 towards Torbay, turning onto A3022 and then right onto A379: take B3205 to Kingswear and Dartmouth ferry: site is close to ferry landing and Royal Dart Y.C.
Waters accessed:	River Dart and Start Bay

Brixham Harbour - Breakwater Slipway
Tel: (01803) 853321 (Harbour Master)

Type:	steep concrete slipway
Suits:	all craft except pwc
Availability:	all states of tide
Restrictions:	5 knot speed limit in harbour: no pwc; water-skiing and windsurfing prohibited in harbour; access road is narrow
Facilities:	diesel from Brixham Marina, petrol from garage nearby, parking for car and trailer (c), toilets on site, chandlery in nearby marina, diving supplies and outboard repairs in town, cafe
Dues:	none
Charge:	approx. £6
Directions:	from Exeter follow A38/A380 towards Torbay, then A3022 to Brixham Harbour and follow signs to 'Breakwater'
Waters accessed:	Tor Bay

Brixham Harbour - Freshwater Quarry
Tel: (01803) 853321 (Harbour Master)

Type:	steep concrete slipway
Suits:	all craft except pwc
Availability:	all states of tide
Restrictions:	5 knot speed limit in harbour: no pwc; water-skiing and windsurfing prohibited in harbour; access road is narrow
Facilities:	diesel from Brixham Marina, petrol from garage nearby, parking for car on site and for trailer nearby (c), toilets on quay, chandlery, diving supplies and outboard repairs nearby
Dues:	none
Charge:	approx. £6
Directions:	from Exeter follow A38/A380 towards Torbay, then A3022 to Brixham Harbour and signs to Oxon Cove car park
Waters accessed:	Tor Bay

Brixham Harbour - Oxon Cove
Tel: (01803) 853321 (Harbour Master)

Type:	shallow concrete slipway with locked barrier
Suits:	all craft up to 20'/6.1m LOA except pwc
Availability:	all states of tide
Restrictions:	5 knot speed limit in harbour: no pwc; water-skiing & windsurfing prohibited in harbour; keys to barrier from Harbour Office
Facilities:	diesel from Brixham Marina, petrol from garage nearby, parking for car on site and for trailer nearby (c), toilets on quay, chandlery, diving supplies and outboard repairs nearby
Dues:	none
Charge:	approx. £6

| Directions: | from Exeter follow A38/A380 towards Torbay, then A3022 to Brixham Harbour and for Oxon/Freshwater Cove car parks |
| Waters accessed: | Tor Bay |

Paignton - Harbour Slip

Tel: (01803) 557812 (summer months only)

Type:	shallow concrete ramp onto hard sand
Suits:	all craft up to 24'/7m LOA
Availability:	all states of tide
Restrictions:	5 knot speed limit inshore: water-skiing permitted in designated areas; pwc must be registered with Torbay Council and have proof of insurance
Facilities:	parking for trailer on site and for car nearby, toilets, chandlery, diving supplies, outboard repairs, restaurants all on site
Dues:	included in launching fee
Charge:	approx. £6
Directions:	follow signs from town centre to south end of seafront
Waters accessed:	Tor Bay, Lyme Bay and English Channel

Torquay Harbour - Beacon Quay

Tel: (01803) 292429 (Harbour Master)

Type:	two fairly steep concrete slipways with slippery wooden ends
Suits:	all craft
Availability:	approx. 5 hours either side HW
Restrictions:	5 knot speed limit in harbour and near beaches: water-skiing permitted in designated areas, pwc must be registered with Torbay Council and have proof of insurance
Facilities:	fuel, parking for car and trailer(c), toilets (summer only), chandlery, cafe and outboard repairs all on site; diving supplies nearby
Dues:	included in launching fee
Charge:	approx. £6
Directions:	from Exeter follow A38/A380 towards Torbay, then follow signs to harbour from town centre: site is adjacent Torquay Marina
Waters accessed:	Tor Bay, Lyme Bay and English Channel

Babbacombe Beach

Tel: (01803) 292429 (Harbour Master)

Type:	concrete ramp onto sandy but rocky beach
Suits:	sailing dinghies and small powered craft only: no pwc
Availability:	all states of tide (May to Sept only): notify Beach Master on site before launching
Restrictions:	5 knot speed limit inshore: pwc prohibited; steep one-way single lane access
Facilities:	limited parking for car and trailer on site (c), toilets, pub/restaurant

Dues:	included in launching fee
Charge:	approx. £6
Directions:	follow A38/380 south from Exeter, turning off to Babbacombe
Waters accessed:	Babbacombe Bay, Lyme Bay and English Channel

Shaldon (River Teign) - Albion Street Slipway
Tel: (01626) 773165 (Harbour Office)

Type:	concrete slipway onto shingle
Suits:	dinghies only
Availability:	approx. 4 hours either side HW
Restrictions:	10 mph speed limit in estuary and river and 5 knot speed limit within area marked by yellow buoys off beaches: for water-skiing contact South Devon Water Ski Club Tel: (01626) 873744
Facilities:	toilets, chandlery, diving supplies and outboard repairs all nearby
Dues:	none
Charge:	none
Directions:	from Exeter follow A38/A380 towards Torbay, turning left onto A381 to Teignmouth then right across bridge to Shaldon Fore St and turn left into Albion St
Waters accessed:	Teign Estuary and Babbacombe Bay

Combeinteignhead (River Teign) - Coombe Cellars
Tel: (01626) 773165 (Harbour Office)

Type:	concrete slipway
Suits:	dinghies and small powered craft
Availability:	approx. 2 hours either side HW
Restrictions:	10 mph speed limit in estuary and river and 5 knot speed limit within area marked by yellow buoys off beaches: for water-skiing contact South Devon Water-Ski Club, Tel: (01626) 873744
Facilities:	parking for car and trailer in pub car park only with permission(c), toilets in pub, chandlery, diving supplies and outboard repairs nearby
Dues:	none
Charge:	none
Directions:	from Exeter follow A38/A380 towards Torbay, turning left onto A381 to Teignmouth then right across bridge to Shaldon; turn immediate right and follow river to Coombe Cellars: site is near Coombe Cellars Inn
Waters accessed:	Teign Estuary and Babbacombe Bay

Teignmouth (River Teign) - Polly Steps Car Park
Tel: (01626) 773165 (Harbour Office)

Type:	concrete slipway
Suits:	all craft up to 20'/6.1m LOA
Availability:	approx. 5 hours either side HW
Restrictions:	10 mph speed limit in estuary and river and 5 knot speed limit within area marked by yellow buoys off

beaches: for water-skiing contact South Devon Water Sports Club, Tel: (01626) 873744; owners/users of all powered craft launching at this site must produce documentary evidence of public liability insurance cover for £1m

Facilities:	fuel nearby, parking for car and trailer on site (c), toilets, chandlery and outboard repairs nearby: this is the best site in Teignmouth
Dues:	none
Charge:	approx. £5 inc. parking
Directions:	from Exeter follow A379 to Teignmouth town centre then signs to Quays along road beside railway line: site is on west side of docks
Waters accessed:	Teign Estuary and Babbacombe Bay

Teignmouth (River Teign) - Gales Hill Slipway

Tel: (01626) 773165 (Harbour Office)

Type:	launching over shingle hard
Suits:	all craft up to approx. 20'/6.1m LOA
Availability:	aapprox. 5 hours either side HW
Restrictions:	10 mph speed limit in estuary and river and 5 knot speed limit within area marked by yellow buoys off beaches: for water-skiing contact South Devon Water-Ski Club, Tel: (01626) 873744
Facilities:	fuel, parking for car (c) and toilets nearby, chandlery from Shaldon
Dues:	none
Charge:	none
Directions:	from Exeter follow A379 to Teignmouth town centre, site is adjacent to quay
Waters accessed:	River Teign and Babbacombe Bay

Exmouth - Foxholes, Seafront

Tel: (01395) 516551 (Water Safety Officer, East Devon District Council)

Type:	steep concrete slipway onto soft dry sand
Suits:	pwc only - craft must be manhandled
Availability:	all states of tide: ramp only gives access onto beach
Restrictions:	buoyed area for pwc: this is only authorised launching site for pwc: 10 knot speed limit in river; do not leave trailers on beach
Facilities:	fuel in town, parking for car and trailer in car park nearby (c), toilets on site, other facilities in town
Dues:	none
Charge:	none
Directions:	from Exeter take A376 to Exmouth then signs to seafront: site is at the E end near the Beach Rescue Centre and opposite the toilets
Waters accessed:	River Exe and Lyme Bay

Exmouth - Imperial Recreation Ground, Royal Avenue

Tel: (01395) 516551 (Water Safety Officer, East Devon District Council)

Type:	wide concrete slipway onto sand/mud
Suits:	sailing craft and small powered craft: no pwc
Availability:	approx. 1 hour either side HW
Restrictions:	10 knot speed limit in river: no pwc permitted to launch from this site: water-skiing permitted outside East Exe buoy
Facilities:	fuel nearby, limited parking for car and trailer on site (c), toilets, windsurfing school, most other facilities in town
Dues:	none
Charge:	none
Directions:	leave M5 at junction 30 following A376 to Exmouth, then follow signs for bus station/sports centre: access is via Royal Avenue
Waters accessed:	River Exe and Lyme Bay

Exmouth - Mamhead Slipway, near the Docks

Tel: (01395) 516551 (Water Safety Officer, East Devon District Council)

Type:	very steep concrete slipway with steel ramp onto sandy beach has sudden drop at end
Suits:	sailing craft and small powered craft: no pwc
Availability:	approx. 2 hours either side HW
Restrictions:	10 knot speed limit in river: pwc are prohibited at this site; site can be congested; water-skiing permitted outside East Exe buoy
Facilities:	fuel (1 mile), limited parking for car and trailer(c), chandlers and diving supplies nearby, toilets nearby, other facilities in town
Dues:	none
Charge:	none
Directions:	leave M5 at junction 30 following A376 to Exmouth, then signs to seafront: site is at west end near Pier and Victoria Road
Waters accessed:	River Exe and Lyme Bay

Lympstone (River Exe) - Sowden End, Sowden Lane

Tel: (01395) 516551 (Water Safety Officer, East Devon District Council)

Type:	concrete slipway onto stone and mud
Suits:	dinghies and sailboards
Availability:	approx. 3 hours either side HW
Restrictions:	10 knot speed limit in river: pwc and powerboats prohibited at this site; narrow access roads
Facilities:	parking for car and trailer nearby (c)
Dues:	none
Charge:	none
Directions:	leave M5 at junction 30 following A376 towards Exmouth and turning off right to Lympstone: access is via Sowden Lane
Waters accessed:	River Exe and Lyme Bay

Budleigh Salterton - Ladram Bay Holiday Centre, Otterton
Tel: (01395) 568398

Type:	concrete slipway onto shingle foreshore
Suits:	dinghies and small powered craft up to 15'/4.6m LOA: no pwc
Availability:	all states of tide with permission
Restrictions:	5 knot speed limit within 200m of shore: water-skiing permitted offshore; pwc prohibited; cars not permitted to drive through caravan park 1000-1800
Facilities:	fuel nearby, parking for car and trailer (c) and toilets on site, pub nearby, boats may be left on beach overnight
Dues:	none
Charge:	dinghies £5, windsurfers/canoes £2; larger boats £10 per day or £40 per week; season tickets (Apr-Oct) available
Directions:	leave M5 at junction 30 following A3052 to Sidmouth; turn left at Newton Poppleford and follow signs to Ladram Bay
Waters accessed:	Lyme Bay

Axmouth Harbour (River Axe)- Seaton Chandlery
Tel: (01297) 24774

Type:	concrete slipway into river north of bridge
Suits:	all craft up to 24'/7.3m LOA
Availability:	approx. 3 hours either side HW by prior arrangement
Restrictions:	5 knot speed limit in river: 8 knot speed limit inshore; water-skiing permitted offshore; entrance to river can be tricky, especially in onshore winds and should only be attempted within 2½ hours HW
Facilities:	diesel on site, petrol nearby, parking for car and trailer (c), toilets and showers, chandlery, moorings, diving supplies and outboard repairs all available on site
Dues:	none
Charge:	approx. £5
Directions:	follow A3052 from Exeter to Seaton: site is adjacent bridge on west side of river
Waters accessed:	River Axe and Lyme Bay

Lyme Regis - The Cobb
Tel: (01297) 442137 (Harbour Master)

Type:	2 shallow wooden and one steeper concrete slipway
Suits:	all craft up to 24'/7.3m LOA except pwc; site is very popular with dive clubs
Availability:	all states of tide
Restrictions:	5 knots in harbour: pwc prohibited; power boats must follow special instructions; access is via a very steep hill with 7.5 ton weight limit

Facilities:	fuel (2 miles), parking for car nearby (c) and trailer on site, toilets and outboard repairs on site, chandlery and diving supplies available nearby; large area at top of slip for rigging/loading etc
Dues:	approx. £7
Charge:	no additional fee
Directions:	follow A35 west from Dorchester and A3052 at Hunters Lodge, two miles east of Axmouth to Lyme Regis
Waters accessed:	Lyme Bay

Bridport Harbour - East Basin

Tel: (0308) 423222 (Harbour Master)

Type:	steep concrete slipway onto wood with 3 tonne weight limit
Suits:	all craft except pwc
Availability:	approx. 3 hours either side HW
Restrictions:	8 knot speed limit: water-skiing permitted 200m from shore but pwc prohibited; slipway is closed by gates during bad weather
Facilities:	fuel (200m), parking for car nearby (c) and for trailers on site, toilets, chandlery, diving supplies, shops and cafe nearby
Dues:	none
Charge:	approx. £5
Directions:	follow A35 west from Dorchester or east from Honiton: at Bridport by-pass, if westbound take 2nd exit at Crown roundabout, if eastbound take 4th exit at Crown roundabout and follow road to car park and slipway
Waters accessed:	Lyme Bay

Weymouth Harbour - Commercial Road Slipway

Tel: (01305) 206423 (Harbour Master)

Type:	shallow concrete ramp
Suits:	all craft up to 22'/6.7m LOA except pwc and wind-surfers
Availability:	all states of tide
Restrictions:	dead slow in harbour: windsurfers, water-skiing and pwc prohibited in harbour; designated zones in Weymouth Bay
Facilities:	diesel from jetty in Outer Harbour, parking for car nearby (c), and for trailer on site, showers in Harbour Office, all other facilities available nearby
Dues:	no separate fee
Charge:	approx. £7 inc. trailer parking
Directions:	from Esplanade roundabout at clock tower, turn right into King St, then left at the bottom, turning into Commercial Rd at the next roundabout: site is opposite multi-storey car park on east side of harbour
Waters accessed:	Weymouth Harbour and Bay

Weymouth - The Beachside Centre, Bowleaze Cove
Tel: (01305) 833216/835562

Type:	long, gentle concrete ramp 16'/5m wide
Suits:	all craft up to 30'/9m LOA
Availability:	approx. 2 hours either side HW or across beach for smaller craft, 1st Apr - 1st Oct: winter launching by prior arrangement
Restrictions:	8 knot speed limit within 250m of shore; all craft launched must carry proof of insurance
Facilities:	parking for car and trailer, toilets, changing rooms, shops, cafe and refreshments
Dues:	none
Charge:	daily launch £12 pwc, £10 dive boats, £8 all other craft: annual permit £145
Directions:	follow brown signs from A353 north of Weymouth Beach
Waters accessed:	Weymouth Bay

Portland (Portland Harbour) - Ferrybridge Marine Services
Tel: (01305) 781518

Type:	concrete slipway
Suits:	all craft
Availability:	all states of tide
Restrictions:	6 knot speed limit in deep water channel: water-skiing and pwc permitted in designated areas
Facilities:	diesel, parking for car and trailer(c) on site ,toilets, chandlery and refreshments, yard facilities, windsurfing and diving supplies all on site
Dues:	on application
Charge:	no separate charge
Directions:	follow signs from Weymouth to Portland (A354), crossing over the Ferry Bridge and taking first left
Waters accessed:	Portland Harbour and Weymouth Bay

Portland (Portland Harbour) - Weymouth & Portland Sailing Academy
Tel: (01305) 860101

Type:	one very large shallow and two large deep-water concrete slipways
Suits:	all craft
Availability:	all states of tide
Restrictions:	6 knot speed limit inshore: visitors must register on arrival
Facilities:	fuel nearby, parking for car and trailer, toilets and showers, clubhouse and bar all on site
Dues:	approx. £2
Charge:	approx. £10 inc. parking and use of club facilities for day
Directions:	follow signs to Portland from Weymouth, along Portland Beach Road, turning left at roundabout into former Air Station: site is located at north end
Waters accessed:	Portland Harbour and Weymouth Bay

Peveril Point, Swanage - Peveril Boat Park, Broad Road

Tel: (01929) 423636

Type:	concrete slipway with winch
Suits:	all craft except pwc
Availability:	all states of tide
Restrictions:	5 knot speed limit inshore: water-skiing permitted off-shore
Facilities:	fuel nearby, parking for car and trailer on site, toilets nearby; chandlery and diving supplies available in town
Dues:	none
Charge:	approx. £13
Directions:	from Poole take A35 and A351 to Swanage following signs for seafront and brown signs to the 'Pier': access is through Broad Road car park
Waters accessed:	Swanage Bay and Durlston Bay

South Coast:
Studland to North Foreland

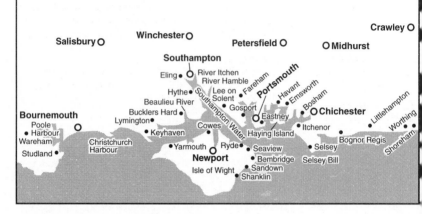

Studland -Shell Bay Marine, Ferry Road
Tel: (01929) 450340

Type:	concrete slipway
Suits:	small powered craft, windsurfers and trailer-sailers
Availability:	approx. 4 hours either side HW by prior arrangement
Restrictions:	speed limit within yellow marker buoys: pwc and water-skiing prohibited; access can be congested and booking is essential
Facilities:	fuel nearby, parking for car and trailer nearby (c), toilets, cafe, moorings, storage and sailing school all on site
Dues:	none
Charge:	approx. £17.50
Directions:	leave Poole on A351 to Swanage, turning off to Studland on B3351: access to site is via toll road to Sandbanks ferry but take immediate left at mini roundabout before entering toll area and go along gravel roadway; from Sandbanks, pay ferry toll,then turn right at mini roundabout and go along gravel road: site is at entrance to Poole Harbour adjacent the Sandbanks/Swanage ferry
Waters accessed:	Poole Harbour and Bay

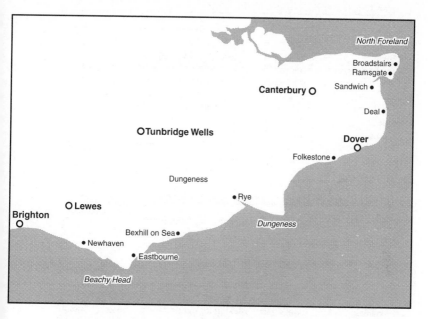

Wareham (River Frome) - Ridge Wharf Yacht Centre
Tel: (01929) 552650 Fax: (01929) 554434

Type:	steep concrete slipway with large winch
Suits:	all craft except pwc (river is narrow for sailing craft)
Availability:	all states of tide except 1 hour either side LW
Restrictions:	4 knot speed limit in river, 10 knots in harbour: water-skiing, pwc and windsurfers prohibited in river
Facilities:	fuel, parking for car and trailer, toilets, chandlery and outboard repairs on site
Dues:	none
Charge:	approx. £7.50 inc. vat and parking
Directions:	follow A351 Swanage road, turning left at roundabout at end of Wareham by-pass: after 300m turn right into New Road and yard is ½ mile ahead
Waters accessed:	River Frome, Poole Harbour and Bay

Wareham (River Frome) - Redclyffe Farm

Tel: (01929) 552225

Type:	shallow concrete ramp
Suits:	all craft except pwc and windsurfers
Availability:	approx. 5 hours either side HW by prior arrangement
Restrictions:	4 knot speed limit in river, 10 knots in harbour: water-skiing, windsurfing and pwc prohibited in river
Facilities:	parking for car and trailer and toilets on site
Dues:	none
Charge:	approx. £7 inc. parking
Directions:	from Poole follow A35/A351 to Wareham, turning off in Stoborough and following signs
Waters accessed:	River Frome, Poole Harbour (1½ miles)

Hamworthy (Poole Harbour) - Rockley Boating Services, Rockley Sands

Tel: (01202) 665001

Type:	concrete slipway
Suits:	all craft
Availability:	all states of tide
Restrictions:	10 knot speed limit in harbour: water-skiing, windsurfing and pwc permitted in designated areas under licence only contact Harbour Office Tel: (01202) 440200
Facilities:	fuel nearby, parking for car and trailer, toilets, chandlery on site
Dues:	only for craft over 15'/4.6m LOA or with engines over 4hp
Charge:	approx. £10.50 inc. parking
Directions:	from Poole follow A350 to Hamworthy, turning off and following signs to Rockley Point
Waters accessed:	Poole Harbour and Bay

Hamworthy (Poole Harbour) - Cobbs Quay, Woodlands Avenue

Tel: (01202) 674299

Type:	long concrete ramp
Suits:	all craft except windsurfers and pwc
Availability:	at all times
Restrictions:	6 knot and 10 knot speed limits in harbour: water-skiing, windsurfing and pwc permitted in designated areas under licence only contact Harbour Office Tel: (01202) 440200; site is above lifting bridge
Facilities:	fuel, parking for car and trailer, toilets, chandlery, outboard repairs, showers and clubhouse all on site
Dues:	only for craft over 15'/4.6m LOA or with engines over 4hp
Charge:	approx. £23.50 (£165 annual)
Directions:	from Poole follow A350 to Hamworthy, turn left by Co-op into Hinchcliffe Rd, and follow signs to Cobbs Quay
Waters accessed:	Poole Harbour above Poole Bridge

Hamworthy (Poole Harbour) - Davis's Boatyard, Cobbs Quay

Tel: (01202) 674349

Type:	shallow concrete ramp
Suits:	all craft except pwc and windsurfers
Availability:	approx. 2 hours either side HW by prior arrangement only
Restrictions:	6 knot and 10 knot speed limits in harbour: water-skiing, windsurfing and pwc permitted in designated areas under licence only contact Harbour Office Tel: (01202) 440200; site is above lifting bridge
Facilities:	fuel nearby, parking for car and trailer and toilets on site, outboard repairs and chandlery nearby
Dues:	only for craft over 15'/4.6m LOA or with engines over 4hp
Charge:	approx. £10 + vat (£68 + vat for season)
Directions:	from Poole follow A350 to Hamworthy, turning left by Co-op into Hinchcliffe Rd, then into Woodlands Ave and Cobbs Quay
Waters accessed:	Poole Harbour above Poole Bridge

Poole (Poole Harbour) - Baiter Public Slipway, Labrador Drive

Tel: (01202) 675151 (Poole Borough Council)

Type:	wide concrete slipway
Suits:	craft up to 21'/6.4m LOA
Availability:	0600 - 2400 hours; approx. 4 hours either side HWS and 5 hours either side HWN
Restrictions:	6 knot and 10 knot speed limits in harbour: water-skiing, windsurfing and pwc permitted in designated areas under licence only, contact Harbour Office Tel: (01202) 440200; car park closes at midnight; site can be very busy
Facilities:	fuel nearby, parking for car and trailer on site; toilets, chandlery and outboard repairs nearby
Dues:	only for craft over 15'/4.6m LOA or with engines over 4hp
Charge:	approx. £5 inc. parking (£3 after 1400 hours): pay at machine in car park
Directions:	from Town Quay follow signs: access is via Newfoundland Drive
Waters accessed:	Poole Harbour and Bay

Sandbanks (Poole Harbour) - Mitchells Boatyard, Turks Lane

Tel: (01202) 747857

Type:	concrete slipway
Suits:	all craft up to 25'/7.6m LOA
Availability:	approx. 1½ hours either side HW by prior arrangement
Restrictions:	6 knot and 10 knot speed limits in harbour: water-skiing, windsurfing and pwc permitted in designated areas under licence only, contact Harbour Office Tel: (01202) 440200; site is very busy in mid-season
Facilities:	fuel (½ mile), limited parking for car and trailer, toilets, chandlery, outboard repairs and yard facilities all on site

Dues:	only for craft over 15'/4.6m LOA or with engines over 4hp
Charge:	approx. £20 inc. parking
Directions:	from Poole town centre follow Sandbanks Rd, turning into Turks Lane after passing Whitecliff recreation ground
Waters accessed:	Poole Harbour and Bay

Lilliput (Poole Harbour) - Salterns Boatyard, 38 Salterns Way

Tel: (01202) 707321

Type:	shallow concrete ramp onto sand; boat hoist and travel hoist
Suits:	all craft
Availability:	all states of tide during working hours by prior arrangement
Restrictions:	6 knot and 10 knot speed limits in harbour: water-skiing, windsurfing and pwc permitted in designated areas under licence only contact Harbour Office Tel: (01202) 440200
Facilities:	fuel, parking for car and trailer, toilets, chandlery, outboard repairs and boatyard facilities all on site; diving supplies nearby
Dues:	only for craft over 15'/4.6m LOA or with engines over 4hp
Charge:	approx. £25.50
Directions:	from Poole town centre follow Sandbanks Rd, turning into Salterns Way
Waters accessed:	Poole Harbour and Bay

Sandbanks (Poole Harbour) - Sandbanks Yacht Co Ltd, 32 Panorama Rd

Tel: (01202) 707500 Fax: (01202) 707575

Type:	shallow concrete ramp
Suits:	all craft up to 22'/6.7m LOA
Availability:	all states of tide except within 1-2 hours LWS
Restrictions:	6 knot and 10 knot speed limits in harbour: water-ski-ing, windsurfing and pwc permitted in designated areas under licence only contact Harbour Office Tel: (01202) 440200
Facilities:	fuel, parking for car and trailer, toilets, chandlery, moorings, repairs and boat storage all available on site
Dues:	only for craft over 15'/4.6m LOA or with engines over 4hp
Charge:	approx. £12.50 inc. parking
Directions:	from Poole town centre follow signs to Sandbanks: Panorama Rd is near Sandbanks ferry
Waters accessed:	Poole Harbour and Bay

Southbourne (River Stour) - Wick Lane

Type:	concrete slipway
Suits:	dinghies and small powered craft
Availability:	approx. 2½ hours either side double HW
Restrictions:	4 knot speed limit in river and harbour: water-skiing and pwc prohibited; currents in harbour entrance are strong
Facilities:	fuel nearby, limited parking for car and trailer (c), toilets on site
Dues:	none
Charge:	none
Directions:	from Bournemouth follow B3059, turning right into Wick Lane before Tuckton Bridge: site is on south bank of river, downstream of bridge
Waters accessed:	River Stour, Christchurch Harbour and Bay

Christchurch (River Stour) - Quomps, Mayors Mead Car Park
Tel: (01202) 495000 (Christchurch Borough Council)

Type:	wide concrete ramp deepens to sudden drop
Suits:	all craft except windsurfers
Availability:	all states of tide except within 1 hour LW
Restrictions:	4 knot speed limit in river and harbour
Facilities:	parking for car and trailer on site (c), toilets nearby
Dues:	none
Charge:	none
Directions:	from Bournemouth follow B3059 towards Christchurch, turning right at roundabout after Tuckton Bridge into Willow Drive: site is adjacent to Wick Ferry and approach is through car park
Waters accessed:	River Stour, Christchurch Harbour and Bay

Christchurch (River Avon) - Rossiter Yachts Ltd. Bridge Street
Tel: (01202) 483250

Type:	concrete slipway
Suits:	all craft except pwc
Availability:	1 hour either side double HW from 0800 -1700 mon-sat, by prior arrangement only
Restrictions:	4 knot speed limit in river and harbour: water-skiing and pwc prohibited
Facilities:	diesel on site, petrol nearby, parking for car and trailer on site, toilets nearby, chandlery and short-stay alongside berths available
Dues:	none
Charge:	approx. £30
Directions:	follow signs to town centre: at roundabout turn into High St and follow into Bridge St; entrance to site is between bridges
Waters accessed:	River Avon leading to Christchurch Harbour and Bay

Christchurch (River Avon) - Bridge Street
Tel: (01202) 495000 (Christchurch Borough Council)

Type:	concrete slipway
Suits:	small powered craft and sailing dinghies only
Availability:	approx. 1 hour either side double HW
Restrictions:	4 knot speed limit in river and harbour
Facilities:	fuel nearby, parking for car on site (c), toilets, chandlery and outboard repairs nearby
Dues:	none
Charge:	none
Directions:	follow B3059 to town centre turning right into Barrack Rd (A35): at roundabout turn into High St and follow into Bridge St: site is on east bank of river adjacent bus turning point and Civic Offices
Waters accessed:	River Avon leading into Christchurch Harbour and Bay

Christchurch (Christchurch Harbour) - Fisherman's Bank, Argyle Road
Tel: (01202) 495000 (Christchurch Borough Council)

Type:	tarmac and shingle foreshore
Suits:	small powered craft and sailing dinghies only
Availability:	approx. 1 hour either side double HW
Restrictions:	4 knot speed limit in harbour: turning and manoeuvring space is very restricted as Argyle Rd is a narrow cul-de-sac
Facilities:	fuel from Stanpit Garage nearby, very limited parking in nearby streets, toilets, chandlers and other facilities available nearby
Dues:	none
Charge:	none
Directions:	from town centre follow B3059 east, turning off to follow signs to Stanpit, turning into Argyle Rd after passing garage
Waters accessed:	Christchurch Harbour and Bay

Mudeford (Christchurch Harbour) - Mudeford Quay
Tel: (01202) 495000 (Christchurch Borough Council)

Type:	concrete ramp onto hard foreshore
Suits:	all craft
Availability:	approx. 1 hour either side double HW
Restrictions:	4 knot speed limit in harbour
Facilities:	fuel from garage (2 miles), parking for car and trailer (c) and toilets on site, other facilities nearby
Dues:	none
Charge:	approx. £3 (hand-launched craft) and £5 (vehicle-launched craft) on summer weekends only
Directions:	from town centre follow B3059 east, turning off to follow signs to Mudeford: access is through car park on Quay
Waters accessed:	Christchurch Harbour and Bay

Keyhaven - The Quay Slipway
Tel: (01590) 645695 (River Warden)

Type:	concrete slipway onto shingle
Suits:	all craft up to 20'/6.1m LOA
Availability:	approx. 3 hours either side HW: launching can be difficult at HWS and impossible an hour either side LW
Restrictions:	4 knot speed limit in estuary and within 300m of shore: water-skiing & pwc prohibited; contact River Warden to discuss suitability of this site for your craft - this is a very restricted site in an environmentally sensitive area
Facilities:	fuel in Milford-on-Sea (1 mile), parking for car and trailer (c), chandlery and outboard repairs on site, toilets nearby
Dues:	approx. £9
Charge:	approx. £9
Directions:	follow A337 to roundabout at New Milton then take B3058 to Milford-on-Sea, following signs to Keyhaven: after passing Gun Inn turn left towards Keyhaven Y.C. and entrance to Quay is ahead
Waters accessed:	Keyhaven Lake and Western Solent

Lymington - Harbour Commissioner's Slip, Town Quay
Tel: (01590) 672014 (Harbour Office)

Type:	wide shallow concrete ramp onto gravel
Suits:	small powered craft except pwc, ski-boats and windsurfers
Availability:	all states of tide
Restrictions:	4 knot advisory speed limit in river: water-skiing, pwc and windsurfing prohibited: access is via narrow and congested road
Facilities:	fuel nearby, limited parking for car (c) and toilets on site; chandlery, outboard repairs, boatyard, shops and pub nearby
Dues:	none
Charge:	approx. £7
Directions:	leave M27 at junction 1 taking A337 to town centre: site is at far end of car park on Town Quay
Waters accessed:	Lymington River and Western Solent

Lymington - Harbour Commissioner's Slip, Bath Road
Tel: (01590) 672014 (Harbour Office)

Type:	wide shallow concrete ramp onto gravel
Suits:	all craft except pwc, ski-boats and windsurfers
Availability:	all states of tide except 1 hour either side LWS
Restrictions:	4 knot advisory speed limit in river: water-skiing, pwc and windsurfing prohibited; take care when ferries approaching
Facilities:	fuel nearby, parking for car, trailer and boat (c) and toilets on site; chandlery, outboard repairs, boatyard, shops and pub nearby

Dues:	none
Charge:	approx. £7
Directions:	leave M27 at junction 1 taking A337 to town centre : site is past Lymington Marina in Bath Road car park
Waters accessed:	Lymington River and Western Solent

Beaulieu River - Bucklers Hard
Tel: (01590) 616200 (Harbour Master)

Type:	concrete slipway
Suits:	all craft except pwc & windsurfers
Availability:	approx. 5 hours either side HW
Restrictions:	5 knot speed limit in river: water-skiing and pwc prohibited
Facilities:	fuel, parking for car and trailer((c) if left for more than 1 day), toilets and chandlery, boatyard, outboard repairs, shop, hotel and maritime museum all on site
Dues:	no separate fee
Charge:	approx. £8 inc. parking
Directions:	leave M27 at junction 1 taking A337 to Lyndhurst then B3056 to Beaulieu following signs to Bucklers Hard; take the third turning left just before Bucklers Hard village
Waters accessed:	Beaulieu River and The Solent

Colwell Bay (Isle of Wight) - Slipway, Colwell Chine
Tel: (01983) 823368 (Isle of Wight Council)

Type:	concrete ramp onto shingle foreshore
Suits:	small craft
Availability:	at all states of tide across beach
Restrictions:	8-10 knot speed limit: locked barrier opened on payment of fee
Facilities:	parking for car (c), toilets and refreshments
Dues:	none
Charge:	approx. £10 registration fee + £2 per day or £35 p.a.
Directions:	follow A3054 west from Newport to Colwell: access to slipway is via Colwell Chine Road
Waters accessed:	Colwell Bay and The Solent

Freshwater Bay (Isle of Wight)
Tel: (01983) 823368 (Isle of Wight Council)

Type:	shingle beach
Suits:	small craft
Availability:	at all staes of tide across beach
Restrictions:	10 knot speed limit inshore: site is used by inshore rescue boat
Facilities:	parking for car and trailer in nearby car park (c), toilets nearby
Dues:	none
Charge:	none
Directions:	follow A3054/5 from Newport: acess to bay is via Military Road
Waters accessed:	Freshwater Bay and English Channel

Yarmouth (Isle of Wight) - Town Quay
Tel: (01983) 760321 (Harbour Office)

Type:	shallow concrete ramp into harbour
Suits:	all craft except windsurfers
Availability:	approx. 2-2½ hours either side HW
Restrictions:	4 knot speed limit in harbour: water-skiing permitted in designated areas in Solent; keep clear of ferries entering and leaving the harbour at all times; access to quay can be restricted by traffic queuing in ferry lanes on quay
Facilities:	fuel on quay, parking for car and trailer (c) nearby, toilets and showers on site, other facilities nearby
Dues:	none
Charge:	none
Directions:	from Cowes follow A3020 and A3054 west to Yarmouth or take ferry across from Lymington
Waters accessed:	Western Solent

Yarmouth (Isle of Wight) - Bridge Road Car Park
Tel: (01983) 760321 (Harbour Office)

Type:	small wooden slipway into river
Suits:	small craft which can be manhandled
Availability:	approx. 2 hours either side HW: soft mud foreshore
Restrictions:	4 knot speed limit in river and harbour; site is above swing bridge
Facilities:	fuel nearby, parking for car, trailer and boat (c), toilets and showers on quay and all other facilities nearby
Dues:	none
Charge:	none
Directions:	site is upstream of bridge on east side of river and access is from Bridge Road car park
Waters accessed:	River Yar, Yarmouth Harbour and Western Solent

Gurnard (Isle of Wight) - Shore Road
Tel: (01983) 823367 (Isle of Wight Council)

Type:	concrete slipway
Suits:	small craft and windsurfers only
Availability:	approx. 3 hours either side HW
Restrictions:	8 knot speed limit within 2 miles of Solent beaches
Facilities:	limited parking, trailers can be left by slip, toilets
Dues:	none
Charge:	none
Directions:	from Cowes take A3020 or B3325 west and follow signs to Gurnard: site is adjacent sailing club
Waters accessed:	Western Solent

West Cowes (Isle of Wight) - Egypt Point Slip, The Esplanade
Tel: (01983) 293952 (Harbour Office, Town Quay)

Type:	shallow concrete ramp
Suits:	all craft - popular with pwc and windsurfers
Availability:	approx. 3 hours either side HW

Restrictions:	6 knot speed limit in harbour: water-skiing prohibited; windsurfers must keep clear of the main channel but pwc must keep in the channel to enter and exit the harbour
Facilities:	parking for car and trailer (c), toilets, chandlers and all other facilities in town
Dues:	none
Charge:	none
Directions:	site is at junction of Egypt Hill and the Esplanade
Waters accessed:	River Medina, Cowes Harbour and The Solent

West Cowes (Isle of Wight) - Watch House Slip, Parade

Tel: (01983) 293952 (Harbour Office, Town Quay)

Type:	shallow concrete ramp
Suits:	small powered craft, sailing dinghies and pwc
Availability:	approx. 4 hours either side HW
Restrictions:	6 knot speed limit in harbour: water-skiing prohibited; windsurfers must keep clear of the main channel but pwc must keep in the channel to enter and exit the harbour; access to site may be congested at peak times
Facilities:	fuel nearby, parking for car and trailer nearby (c), most other facilities available in town
Dues:	none
Charge:	none
Directions:	access is from the southern end of the Parade
Waters accessed:	River Medina, Cowes Harbour and the Solent

West Cowes (Isle of Wight) - Sun Hill Slip, High Street

Tel: (01983) 293952 (Harbour Office, Town Quay)

Type:	concrete and stone slipway onto shingle
Suits:	sailing dinghies only
Availability:	approx. 3 hours either side HW: key available 0900 - 1700 from Midland Bank or Harbour Office
Restrictions:	6 knot speed limit in harbour: water-skiing prohibited; windsurfers must keep clear of main channel but pwc must keep within channel to enter and exit harbour; access is via narrow pedestrianised road with a locked barrier
Facilities:	fuel nearby, parking for car and trailer nearby (c), most other facilities available in town
Dues:	none
Charge:	none
Directions:	site is off High St, adjacent Midland Bank and opposite Sun Hill
Waters accessed:	River Medina, Cowes Harbour and the Solent

West Cowes (Isle of Wight) - Thetis Wharf, Medina Road
Tel: (01983) 293952 (Harbour Office, Town Quay)

Type:	shallow concrete ramp onto shingle
Suits:	sailing dinghies only
Availability:	approx. 4 hours either side HW
Restrictions:	6 knot speed limit in harbour: water-skiing prohibited; windsurfers must keep clear of main channel but pwc must keep in the channel to enter and exit harbour
Facilities:	fuel nearby, parking for car and trailer nearby (c), most other facilities available in town
Dues:	none
Charge:	none
Directions:	from town centre, follow directions to Floating Bridge: site is opposite Bridge Rd at northern end of Medina Rd
Waters accessed:	River Medina, Cowes Harbour and the Solent

East Cowes (Isle of Wight) - White Hart Slip, Dover Road
Tel: (01983) 293952 (Harbour Office, Town Quay)

Type:	narrow concrete slipway
Suits:	sailing dinghies only
Availability:	approx. 4 hours either side HW
Restrictions:	6 knot speed limit in harbour: water-skiing prohibited; windsurfers must keep clear of main channel but pwc must keep in channel to enter and exit harbour
Facilities:	fuel nearby, parking for car and trailer nearby (c), most other facilities available in town
Dues:	none
Charge:	none
Directions:	site is adjacent Red Funnel Ferry Terminal and vehicular access is restricted
Waters accessed:	River Medina, Cowes Harbour and the Solent

East Cowes (Isle of Wight) - Albany Road
Tel: (01983) 293952 (Harbour Office, Town Quay)

Type:	short, stepped masonry slipway
Suits:	small craft which can be manhandled only
Availability:	HW only
Restrictions:	6 knot speed limit in harbour: water-skiing prohibited; windsurfers must keep clear of main channel but pwc must keep in channel to enter and exit harbour
Facilities:	parking for car and trailer, toilets
Dues:	none
Charge:	none
Directions:	access is via the Esplanade
Waters accessed:	River Medina, Cowes Harbour and the Solent

Newport (Isle of Wight) - Old Town Quay
Tel: (01983) 525994 (Harbour Office)

Type:	shallow concrete ramp
Suits:	all craft up to 20'/6.1m LOA
Availability:	approx. 2 hours either side HW
Restrictions:	4 knot speed limit in river and harbour: site is on corner of busy road with no pavement; Seaclose Quay is a better site
Facilities:	parking for car & trailer on site, toilets nearby
Dues:	none
Charge:	none
Directions:	from Cowes follow A3020 or from Ryde the A3054: site is at the junction of Sea St with the Town Quay
Waters accessed:	River Medina and the Solent

Newport (Isle of Wight) - Seaclose Quay
Tel: (01983) 525994 (Harbour Office)

Type:	steep concrete ramp
Suits:	all craft up to 20'/6.1m LOA
Availability:	approx. 2 hours either side HW
Restrictions:	4 knot speed limit in river and harbour: care needed`as site is close to entrance of large transport yard which must not be obstructed
Facilities:	parking for car & trailer on site, toilets nearby; this is the best site in Newport
Dues:	none
Charge:	none
Directions:	from Cowes follow A3020 or from Ryde the A3054: site is reached via the Town Quay and is 500m south of previous site
Waters accessed:	River Medina, Cowes Harbour and the Solent

Newport (Isle of Wight) - Island Harbour Marina, Mill Lane
Tel: (01983) 822999

Type:	concrete slipway into locked marina basin
Suits:	all craft up to 50'/15m LOA
Availability:	approx. 4 hours either side HW by prior arrangement
Restrictions:	4 knot speed limit in river and harbour
Facilities:	diesel on site, petrol nearby, parking for car and trailer, toilets, showers (c), engine repairs, launderette, boat-building, overnight berths, pub and restaurant facilities
Dues:	none
Charge:	approx. £30
Directions:	from Newport or Ryde follow A3054 turning off into Fairlee Rd: site is on east bank of river downstream of Newport
Waters accessed:	River Medina, Cowes Harbour and the Solent

Whippingham (Isle of Wight) - The Folly Inn, Folly Road

Type:	shallow concrete ramp
Suits:	all craft
Availability:	approx. 2 hours either side HW: site is not useable for an hour either side of HW
Restrictions:	6 knot speed limit in Folly Reach
Facilities:	fuel nearby, parking for car and trailer in field only, pub with toilets and showers (0900-2300) and restaurant facilities, chandlery and outboard repairs nearby
Dues:	none
Charge:	none
Directions:	from Newport or Ryde follow A3054 turning off into Folly Lane: site is on east bank of river, upstream of East Cowes and access is through The Folly Inn car park
Waters accessed:	River Medina, Cowes Harbour and The Solent

Ryde (Isle of Wight) - St Thomas' Street

Tel: (01983) 613879 (Harbour Master): Ryde Rescue Tel: (01983) 564564

Type:	shallow concrete ramp onto beach
Suits:	small craft only
Availability:	approx. 3 hours either side HW
Restrictions:	6 knot speed limit inshore; narrow access between houses to site - harbour slipway (next entry) is better site
Facilities:	fuel, parking for car and trailer (c) and toilets all nearby
Dues:	none
Charge:	none
Directions:	site is to the west of pier
Waters accessed:	The Solent

Ryde (Isle of Wight) - Harbour Slipway

Tel: (01983) 613879 (Harbour Master): Ryde Rescue Tel: (01983) 564564

Type:	shallow concrete ramp
Suits:	all craft
Availability:	approx. 3 hours either side HW
Restrictions:	6 knot speed limit inshore
Facilities:	fuel from nearby garage, parking for car and trailer (c) and toilets on site, outboard repairs available through Harbour Office
Dues:	none
Charge:	none
Directions:	site is east of pier at harbour and access is from the Esplanade, adjacent to the Pavilion
Waters accessed:	The Solent

Ryde (Isle of Wight) - Appley Slip, Northwalk

Tel: (01983) 613879 (Harbour Master): Ryde Rescue Tel: (01983) 564564

Type:	shingle foreshore onto sandy beach
Suits:	small craft which can be manhandled only
Availability:	approx. 3 hours either side HW
Restrictions:	6 knot speed limit inshore
Facilities:	fuel nearby, parking for car and trailer (c) and toilets on site
Dues:	none
Charge:	none
Directions:	site is at the east end of Northwalk at Appley Park next to Ryde Rowing Club: Ryde Rescue operates from this site
Waters accessed:	The Solent

Seaview (Isle of Wight) - Crown Slip

Tel: (01983) 823368 (Isle of Wight Council)

Type:	concrete/stone ramp onto shingle and sand beach
Suits:	small craft only
Availability:	at all states of tide across beach
Restrictions:	speed limit inshore
Facilities:	parking for car, toilets, chandlery and outboard repairs all nearby
Dues:	none
Charge:	none
Directions:	from Ryde follow B3330 and signs to Seaview: site is accessed from Bluett Avenue
Waters accessed:	The Solent

Seaview (Isle of Wight)- Esplanade

Tel: (01983) 823368 (Isle of Wight Council)

Type:	very steep concrete slipway with sharp bend onto shingle
Suits:	small craft only
Availability:	approx. 3 hours either side HW
Restrictions:	6 knot speed limit inshore
Facilities:	none on site
Dues:	none
Charge:	none
Directions:	from Ryde follow B3330 and signs to Seaview and seafront: site is at junction of High St and Esplanade on sharp bend
Waters accessed:	The Solent

Seagrove Bay (Isle of Wight) - Pier Road

Tel: (01983) 823368 (Isle of Wight Council)

Type:	concrete slipway onto hard sandy beach
Suits:	small craft only
Availability:	at all states of tide across the beach
Restrictions:	speed limit inshore

Facilities:	toilets nearby
Dues:	none
Charge:	none
Directions:	from Ryde follow Easthill Rd, Eddington Rd, Seaview Lane, Old Seaview Lane and then into Pier Rd
Waters accessed:	The Solent

Seagrove Bay (Isle of Wight) - Gully Road

Tel: (01983) 823368 (Isle of Wight Council)

Type:	concrete slipway onto sandy beach
Suits:	small craft only
Availability:	at all states of tide across beach
Restrictions:	speed limit inshore: no space for parking
Facilities:	toilets
Dues:	none
Charge:	none
Directions:	from Ryde follow Easthill Rd, Calthorpe Rd, Nettlestone Hill, Priory Drive and Gully Rd: site is at southern end of bay
Waters accessed:	The Solent

St Helens Duver (Isle of Wight)

Tel: (01983) 823368 (Isle of Wight Council)

Type:	shallow concrete ramp onto sandy beach
Suits:	all craft
Availability:	approx. 2½ hours either side HW or at all states of tide across beach
Restrictions:	speed limit inshore
Facilities:	parking for car and trailer (c), toilets and cafe all on site
Dues:	none
Charge:	none
Directions:	from Ryde follow B3330 to St Helens and signs to 'The Duver': access is through car park and site is adjacent to old church
Waters accessed:	The Solent

St Helens Duver (Isle of Wight) - H. Attrill & Sons (IOW) Ltd

Tel: (01983) 872319

Type:	concrete slipway
Suits:	all craft except pwc: craft over 20'/6.1m LOA launched by yard staff only
Availability:	approx. 3 hours either side HW
Restrictions:	6 knot speed limit in harbour: no water-skiing or wind-surfing; tides in harbour entrance run very strongly
Facilities:	diesel, parking for car and trailer (c), boatyard, other facilities nearby
Dues:	none
Charge:	approx. £19 for craft under 20'/6.1m LOA

Directions:	from Ryde follow B3330 to St Helens then road across The Duver
Waters accessed:	Bembridge Harbour and The Solent

Bembridge Harbour - Bembridge Outboards, Embankment Rd
Tel: (01983) 872817

Type:	medium concrete ramp
Suits:	all craft except pwc and windsurfers
Availability:	approx. 2½ hours either side HW; contact owners to ensure site will not be obstructed
Restrictions:	6 knot speed limit in harbour; windsurfing and water-skiing prohibited; tide in harbour entrance runs very strongly
Facilities:	diesel nearby, petrol (2 miles), parking for car and trailer nearby, toilets available during working hours, outboard repairs and boat sales on site, chandlers nearby
Dues:	none
Charge:	approx. £2
Directions:	take A3055 and B3330 from Ryde: access is via Embankment Rd on the southern shore of the harbour
Waters accessed:	Bembridge Harbour and the Solent

Bembridge Harbour (Isle of Wight) - Wades Pontoon, Embankment Rd
Tel: (01983) 872828 (Harbour Office)

Type:	moderate concrete ramp onto rough ground
Suits:	small sailing and powered craft
Availability:	approx. 2½ hours either side HW by prior arrangement
Restrictions:	6 knot speed limit in harbour: water-skiing and wind-surfing prohibited; tides in harbour entrance run very strongly
Facilities:	fuel nearby, no parking, toilets, chandlery and diving supplies nearby, outboard repairs from Bembridge Outboards adjacent
Dues:	none
Charge:	none
Directions:	take A3055 and B3330 from Ryde: access is from Embankment Rd between A.A. Coombes and Bembridge Outboards
Waters accessed:	Bembridge Harbour and the Solent

Bembridge Harbour (Isle of Wight) - A.A.Coombes, Embankment Rd
Tel: (01983) 872296

Type:	concrete slipway
Suits:	all craft except pwc
Availability:	approx. 2 hours either side HW: contact yard to ensure site will be available
Restrictions:	6 knot speed limit in harbour: water-skiing and wind-surfing prohibited; tides in harbour entrance run very strongly

Facilities:	diesel on site, petrol (2 miles), parking for car and trailer (c) and toilets nearby, chandlery, boat repairs, storage, moorings all available on site; outboard repairs from Bembridge Outboards adjacent
Dues:	none
Charge:	approx. £2
Directions:	take A3055 and B3330 from Ryde: site is on Embankment Rd which runs around harbour from St Helens to Bembridge village
Waters accessed:	Bembridge Harbour and the Solent

Shanklin (Isle of Wight) - Palestine Slipway, The Esplanade

Tel: (01983) 823368 (Isle of Wight Council)

Type:	shallow concrete ramp onto sand/shingle beach
Suits:	small sailing and powered craft
Availability:	at all times across beach
Restrictions:	10 knot speed limit inshore: locked barrier to site
Facilities:	parking for car and trailer and toilets nearby, refreshments
Dues:	none
Charge:	£10 registration, then £2 (inc. parking) per day (£25 p.a.)
Directions:	in Shanklin, follow Esplanade south from Pier to end
Waters accessed:	English Channel

Shanklin (Isle of Wight) - Hope Beach

Tel: (01983) 823368 (Isle of Wight Council)

Type:	concrete ramp onto sand and shingle beach
Suits:	small sailing and powered craft
Availability:	at all times across beach
Restrictions:	10 knot speed limit inshore
Facilities:	parking for car on site and for trailer nearby (c), toilets nearby, refreshments
Dues:	none
Charge:	none
Directions:	site is at north end of Shanklin seafront, at the junction of Hope Road and the Esplanade and adjacent to the car park
Waters accessed:	English Channel

Sandown (Isle of Wight) - Yaverland

Tel: (01983) 823368 (Isle of Wight Council)

Type:	concrete slipway onto hard sand beach
Suits:	small craft
Availability:	at all states of tide across the beach
Restrictions:	speed limit inshore
Facilities:	parking for car and trailer (c) at sailing club with permission, toilets
Dues:	none
Charge:	none

| Directions: | access is via Sandown High Street and Yaverland Rd: site is adjacent Sailing Club |
| Waters accessed: | English Channel |

Sandown (Isle of Wight) - Avenue Slipway
Tel: (01983) 823368 (Isle of Wight Council)

Type:	stone slipway onto soft sandy beach
Suits:	small sailing craft
Availability:	at all states of tide across beach
Restrictions:	speed limit inshore
Facilities:	limited parking on street, toilets, refreshments
Dues:	none
Charge:	none
Directions:	from Sandown High Street take Esplanade Rd onto the Esplanade: site is adjacent to Eastern Gardens
Waters accessed:	English Channel

Sandown (Isle of Wight) - Devonia
Tel: (01983) 823368 (Isle of Wight Council)

Type:	concrete slipway onto soft sandy beach
Suits:	small craft
Availability:	at all states of tide across beach
Restrictions:	speed limit inshore
Facilities:	limited parking on street only, toilets and refreshments
Dues:	none
Charge:	none
Directions:	follow Sandown High Street to Pier St and the Esplanade
Waters accessed:	English Channel

Calshot Spit, Fawley - Calshot Activities Centre
Tel: (02380) 892077

Type:	steep concrete ramp
Suits:	all craft: assisted launch available by prior arrangement
Availability:	at all states of tide except 1 hour either side LWS from 0800 -2200
Restrictions:	4 knot speed limit within100m shore; water-skiing prohibited; do not obstruct dinghy sailers under tuition; site is very close to main shipping channel and all craft must have 3rd party insurance
Facilities:	fuel (2 miles), parking for car and trailer, toilets and showers, bar and cafe, boat park, storage for craft up to 40'/12.2m LOA and accommodation all available on site
Dues:	none
Charge:	approx. £8.50 inc. vat, parking and use of facilties
Directions:	from Southampton take the A326 to Fawley then B3053 to Calshot Spit and Castle
Waters accessed:	Southampton Water and Solent

Fawley (Southampton Water) - Public Hard, Ashlett Creek

Type:	shingle hard
Suits:	sailing dinghies and trailer-sailers
Availability:	approx. 3 hours either side HW
Restrictions:	6 knot speed limit: no water-skiing or pwc; narrow access road
Facilities:	limited parking for car and trailer on site, toilets nearby, pub
Dues:	none
Charge:	none
Directions:	from Southampton take the A326 to Fawley then B3053 and turn off to Ashlett
Waters accessed:	Southampton Water

Hythe (Southampton Water) - Hythe Marina Village, Shamrock Way
Tel. (023) 8020 7073

Type:	wide (40'/12.2m) steep concrete ramp
Suits:	all craft except windsurfers and pwc
Availability:	approx. 2 hours either side HW
Restrictions:	6 knot speed limit north of slipway: no windsurfing, water-skiing or pwc; access road has speed ramps
Facilities:	fuel, parking for car and trailer, toilets, telephone, chandlery, pub, shop and all marina facilities are adjacent
Dues:	none
Charge:	none
Directions:	leave M27 westbound taking M271 and following signs for Totton/Lyndhurst; pick up A326 (signposted to Fawley) and follow signs for Hythe village centre and marina
Waters accessed:	Southampton Water and the Solent

Marchwood (River Test) - Cracknore Hard
Tel: (023) 8048 8665 (Harbour Master)

Type:	wide rather soft shingle hard
Suits:	small craft which can be manhandled only
Availability:	approx. 4 hours either side HW
Restrictions:	6 knot speed limit: water-skiing permitted in designated area in River Test; access is narrow and rough - this is a poor site
Facilities:	no facilities apart from very limited parking
Dues:	none
Charge:	none
Directions:	from Southampton follow A35 to Rushington roundabout, taking Marchwood by-pass and turning left into Jacobgutter Lane to follow signs to 'Cracknore Hard'
Waters accessed:	River Test, Southampton Water and the Solent

Marchwood (River Test) - Magazine Lane
Tel: (023) 8048 8665 (Harbour Master)

Type:	shallow shingle hard
Suits:	craft up to about 15'/4.6m LOA
Availability:	approx. 4 hours either side HW
Restrictions:	6 knot speed limit: water-skiing permitted in designated area in River Test; access is narrow and rough and turning and parkingspace very limited
Facilities:	limited parking for car and trailer on site: Marchwood Y.C.adjacent
Dues:	none
Charge:	none
Directions:	follow A35 from Southampton to Rushington round-about, taking Marchwood by-pass and turning left into Jacobgutter Lane towards Marchwood. At roundabout take Normandy Way and Magazine Lane is second road on left
Waters accessed:	River Test, Southampton Water and The Solent

Eling Creek (River Test) - Eling Quay
Tel: (023) 8086 3138

Type:	shingle hard with drop at end onto mud
Suits:	all craft
Availability:	approx. 2 hours either side HW
Restrictions:	6 knot speed limit: water-skiing permitted in designated area in River Test; parking space can be congested
Facilities:	parking for car and trailer on site , toilets nearby, cafe and pub
Dues:	none
Charge:	none
Directions:	from the M27 take the A271 and A35 west following signs to Eling Tide Mill: site is adjacent Anchor Inn and Tide Mill Visitor Centre
Waters accessed:	Southampton Water and The Solent

Southampton (River Test) - Town Quay

Type:	steep wide (15'/4.6m) concrete ramp
Suits:	all trailed craft
Availability:	approx. 2 hours either side HW
Restrictions:	6 knot speed limit: water-skiing permitted in designated area in River Test
Facilities:	fuel from marina, parking for car and trailer (c)
Dues:	none
Charge:	none
Directions:	site is adjacent to Town Quay Marina and access is through car park
Waters accessed:	River Test, Southampton Water and The Solent

Southampton, Chapel (River Itchen) - Crosshouse Hard

Tel: (023) 8083 3605 (Local Services, Southampton City Council)

Type:	wide concrete slipway onto muddy shore
Suits:	small shallow-draught craft
Availability:	approx. 5 hours either side HW
Restrictions:	6 knot speed limit: water-skiing permitted in designated area in River Test
Facilities:	parking for car and trailer nearby (c) but not overnight
Dues:	none
Charge:	none
Directions:	site is on west side of river just north of the Itchen Bridge: access is via Crosshouse Rd
Waters accessed:	River Itchen, Southampton Water and The Solent

Southampton, Chapel (River Itchen) - Belvedere Wharf

Tel: (023) 8083 3605 (Local Services, Southampton City Council)

Type:	concrete slipway and gravel hard
Suits:	small shallow-draught craft only
Availability:	at all states of tide except 1 hour either side LW
Restrictions:	6 knot speed limit: water-skiing permitted in designated area in River Test
Facilities:	fuel nearby, limited parking for car and trailer, chandlery nearby
Dues:	none
Charge:	none
Directions:	from city centre, follow signs to Bitterne, then Northam Rd, Redcliffe Rd, Union Rd, Princes St, Millbank St: access to site is via Belvedere Rd
Waters accessed:	River Itchen, Southampton Water and The Solent

Southampton, Northam (River Itchen) - Old Mill Quay

Tel: (023) 8083 3605 (Local Services, Southampton City Council)

Type:	concrete slipway and gravel hard
Suits:	small shallow-draught craft
Availability:	at all states of tide except 1 hour either side LW
Restrictions:	6 knot speed limit: water-skiing permitted in designated area in River Test
Facilities:	fuel from garage, parking for car and trailer nearby, chandlery nearby
Dues:	none
Charge:	none
Directions:	from city centre, follow signs to Bitterne, then Northam Rd, Redcliffe Rd, Union Rd: access to site is via Princes St
Waters accessed:	River Itchen, Southampton Water and The Solent

Southampton, St Denys (River Itchen) - Priory Hard
Tel: (023) 8083 3605 (Local Services, Southampton City Council)

Type:	concrete slipway and gravel hard
Suits:	small shallow-draught craft
Availability:	approx. 5 hours either side HW
Restrictions:	6 knot speed limit: water-skiing permitted in designated area in River Test
Facilities:	fuel from garage, limited parking for car and trailer
Dues:	none
Charge:	none
Directions:	from city centre follow signs to St Denys Station: site is on west side of river south of the station and access is via Priory Rd
Waters accessed:	River Itchen, Southampton Water and The Solent

Southampton, Woolston (River Itchen) - Nuns Walk
Tel: (023) 8083 3605 (Local Services, Southampton City Council)

Type:	steep shingle shore
Suits:	canoes and windsurfers
Availability:	at all states of tide except 1 hour either side LW
Restrictions:	6 knot speed limit: water-skiing permitted in designated area in River Test
Facilities:	parking for car only nearby
Dues:	none
Charge:	none
Directions:	leave M27 at junction 8 and follow A3025 to Woolston or from city centre cross Itchen Bridge: site is on east side of river just north of the bridge and access is via Hazel Rd
Waters accessed:	River Itchen, Southampton Water and The Solent

Southampton, Woolston (River Itchen) - Itchen Ferry Hard
Tel: (023) 8083 3605 (Local Services, Southampton City Council)

Type:	concrete slipway
Suits:	small shallow-draught craft
Availability:	approx. 5 hours either side HW
Restrictions:	6 knot speed limit: water-skiing permitted in designated area in River Test
Facilities:	parking for car and trailer on street only, chandlery nearby
Dues:	none
Charge:	none
Directions:	leave M27 at junction 8 and follow A3025 to Woolston or from city centre cross Itchen Bridge: site is on east side of river just north of the bridge and access is via Hazel Rd
Waters accessed:	River Itchen, Southampton Water and The Solent

Southampton, Woolston (River Itchen) - Floating Bridge Hard

Type:	concrete slipway
Suits:	all trailed craft
Availability:	most states of tide
Restrictions:	6 knot speed limit: water-skiing permitted in designated area in River Test
Facilities:	parking for car and trailer
Dues:	none
Charge:	none
Directions:	leave M27 at junction 8 and follow A3025 to Woolston or from city centre cross Itchen Bridge: site is on east side of river south of the Itchen Bridge
Waters accessed:	River Itchen, Southampton Water and The Solent

Southampton, Weston Point (River Itchen) - Victoria Road Slipway

Tel: (023) 8083 3605 (Local Services, Southampton City Council)

Type:	concrete slipway with central wooden skid
Suits:	small craft and craft with keels up to approx. 20'/6.1m LOA
Availability:	approx. 5 hours either side HW
Restrictions:	6 knot speed limit: water-skiing permitted in designated area of River Test
Facilities:	parking for car and trailer
Dues:	none
Charge:	none
Directions:	leave M27 at junction 8 and follow A3025 to Woolston or from city centre cross Itchen Bridge: site is on east side of river south of the bridge and adjacent Southampton S.C. clubhouse; access is via Victoria Rd at junction with Swift Road
Waters accessed:	River Itchen, Southampton Water and The Solent

Weston (Southampton Water) - Weston Hard, Weston Lane

Tel: (023) 8083 3605 (Local Services, Southampton City Council)

Type:	slipway with central wooden skid
Suits:	small craft
Availability:	approx. 5 hours either side HW
Restrictions:	6 knot speed limit: water-skiing permitted in designated area in River Test
Facilities:	parking for car and trailer (not overnight)
Dues:	none
Charge:	none
Directions:	leave M27 at junction 8 and follow A3025 turning off to Weston: site is at end of Weston Lane and access is via Weston Parade
Waters accessed:	Southampton Water and The Solent

Netley Abbey (Southampton Water) - Beach Lane Slipway
Tel: (023) 8045 3732 (Hound P.C.)

Type:	concrete slipway onto shingle
Suits:	small craft
Availability:	approx. 2 hours either side HW by prior arrangement
Restrictions:	6 knot speed limit: water-skiing permitted in designated areas; site only available if boat is kept in compound (c) - contact number above for further information
Facilities:	fuel in village, parking for car and trailer, boat compound, toilets
Dues:	none
Charge:	on application
Directions:	leave M27 at junction 8 and follow A3025, turning off to Netley Abbey: site is approached via Victoria Rd
Waters accessed:	Southampton Water and The Solent

Hamble (River Hamble) - Hamble Quay, High Street
Tel: (01489) 576387 (Harbour Office)

Type:	shallow concrete ramp
Suits:	all craft up to approx. 24'/7.3m LOA except ski-boats, windsurfers and pwc
Availability:	approx. 1½ hours either side HW
Restrictions:	vessels must not cause wash: water-skiing and windsurfing prohibited in river; pwc should launch at Warsash Hard; popular and busy site with narrow and congested access
Facilities:	fuel in village or at local marinas, limited parking for car and trailer (c), toilets, chandlery and outboard repairs nearby
Dues:	none
Charge:	none
Directions:	leave M27 at junction 8 and follow B3397 to Hamble: site is at end of High St adjacent Royal Southern Y.C. and opposite the Bugle Inn
Waters accessed:	River Hamble, Southampton Water and The Solent

Hamble (River Hamble) - Port Hamble Marina
Tel: (023) 8045 4111 (Hamble Yacht Services)

Type:	concrete slipway
Suits:	larger craft only
Availability:	all states of tide by prior arrangement
Restrictions:	vessels must not cause wash: water-skiing and windsurfing prohibited in river
Facilities:	fuel, limited parking for car and trailer, toilets, showers, chandlery and other marina facilities all on site
Dues:	none
Charge:	min. charge £59
Directions:	leave M27 at junction 8 and follow B3397 to Hamble and then signs to marina
Waters accessed:	River Hamble, Southampton Water and The Solent

Hamble (River Hamble) - Mercury Yacht Harbour, Satchell Lane
Tel: (023) 8045 5994

Type:	concrete slipway
Suits:	all craft except ski-boats
Availability:	approx. 3 hours either side HW
Restrictions:	vessels must not cause wash: water-skiing and windsurfing prohibited in river
Facilities:	fuel nearby, parking for car and trailer, toilets and showers, chandlery and other marina facilities all on site
Dues:	none
Charge:	approx. £12
Directions:	leave M27 at junction 8 and follow B3397 to Hamble and then signs to yacht harbour
Waters accessed:	River Hamble, Southampton Water and The Solent

Bursledon (River Hamble) - Lands End Road
Tel: (01489) 576387 (Harbour Office)

Type:	shingle foreshore
Suits:	dinghies only: pwc should launch from Warsash Hard
Availability:	approx. 4-5 hours either side HW
Restrictions:	vessels must not make wash: water-skiing and windsurfing prohibited in river
Facilities:	fuel nearby, parking at station (1/2 mile), pub, chandlery nearby
Dues:	none
Charge:	none
Directions:	leave M27 at junction 8 and follow A27 to Bursledon, turning right in village towards Bursledon Pt: site is opposite Moody's Boatyard and close to "Jolly Sailor" pub
Waters accessed:	River Hamble, Southampton Water and The Solent

Lower Swanwick (River Hamble) - Swanwick Shore Road Hard
Tel: (01489) 576387 (Harbour Office)

Type:	shingle hard
Suits:	small craft except pwc
Availability:	approx. 4-5 hours either side HW
Restrictions:	vessels must not make wash: water-skiing and windsurfing prohibited in river; pwc should launch at Warsash (next site)
Facilities:	fuel and limited parking nearby, chandlery from marina
Dues:	none
Charge:	none
Directions:	leave M27 at junction 9 and follow A27: site is on east bank of river, just downstream of Moody's Marina
Waters accessed:	River Hamble, Southampton Water and The Solent

Warsash (River Hamble) - Shore Road Hard
Tel: (01489) 576387 (Harbour Office)

Type:	shingle hard
Suits:	all craft: best site for pwc
Availability:	all states of tide
Restrictions:	6 knot speed limit: water-skiing prohibited in river but good access to designated areas in Southampton Water; this is the recommended site for launching pwc in the river
Facilities:	fuel, limited parking for car and trailer, toilets, chandlery and outboard repairs all nearby, pub
Dues:	none
Charge:	none
Directions:	leave A27 at Park Gate via Brook Lane following signs for Warsash and turning right along Shore Rd: site is on east bank of river near mouth and opposite 'The Rising Sun' pub
Waters accessed:	River Hamble, Southampton Water and The Solent

Hill Head - Salterns Road

Type:	timber ramp onto shingle beach
Suits:	sailing dinghies and windsurfers
Availability:	approx. 4 hours either side HW
Restrictions:	10 knot speed limit within 100m of shore: water-skiing prohibited except within designated areas; popular and busy site
Facilities:	parking for car and trailer on site (c), toilets and chandlery nearby
Dues:	none
Charge:	none
Directions:	turn off the A27 west of Fareham into B3334 Stubbington Lane following signs to Hill Head; site is at end of large car park near Seafarers S.C.
Waters accessed:	The Solent

Hill Head- site adjacent Hill Head S.C.
Tel. (01329) 664843 (Hill Head S.C.)

Type:	steep wooden ramp
Suits:	sailing dinghies and windsurfers
Availability:	approx. 2 hours either side HW
Restrictions:	speed limit inshore: narrow access through car park
Facilities:	parking for car and trailer, chandlery nearby, Hill Head S.C. adjacent
Dues:	none
Charge:	none
Directions:	follow A27 west of Fareham into B3334 Stubbington Lane following signs to Hill Head
Waters accessed:	The Solent

Lee-on-Solent - HMS Daedalus Slipway, Marine Parade West

Type:	concrete ramp
Suits:	all trailed craft especially ski-boats and pwc
Availability:	at all states of tide
Restrictions:	speed limit inshore
Facilities:	limited parking for car and trailer, toilets nearby
Dues:	none
Charge:	none
Directions:	follow B3333 to Lee-on-Solent: site is at western end of seafront
Waters accessed:	The Solent

Lee-on-Solent - Marine Parade East
Tel: (023) 9258 4242 (Leisure Division, Gosport Borough Council)

Type:	steep concrete slipway
Suits:	all craft
Availability:	approx. 4 hours either side HW
Restrictions:	speed limit inshore: water-skiing permitted in designated area
Facilities:	parking for car and trailer (c), toilets, chandlery from Gosport
Dues:	none
Charge:	none
Directions:	leave M27 at junction11 following A27 then B3385 to seafront
Waters accessed:	The Solent

Lee-on-Solent - Sailing Club, Marine Parade East
Tel: (023) 9258 4242 (Leisure Division, Gosport Borough Council)

Type:	concrete slipway onto shingle
Suits:	all craft
Availability:	approx. 2½ hours either side HW or over shingle at all times
Restrictions:	7 knot speed limit within 1km of beach: water-skiing permitted in designated area
Facilities:	parking for car and trailer (c), toilets, chandlery from Gosport
Dues:	none
Charge:	none
Directions:	leave M27 at junction11 following A27 then B3385 to seafront
Waters accessed:	The Solent

Stokes Bay - No. 2 Battery
Tel: (023) 9258 4242 (Leisure Division, Gosport Borough Council)

Type:	3 concrete slipways: best one is at No 2 battery
Suits:	all craft
Availability:	approx. 4 hours either side HW or over shingle at all times

Restrictions:	speed limit inshore: water-skiing permitted in designated area
Facilities:	parking for car and trailer (c), toilets, chandlery from Gosport
Dues:	none
Charge:	none
Directions:	leave M27 at junction11 and follow A27 then B3385/B3333 to seafront: site is at west end of Stokes Bay Road
Waters accessed:	The Solent

Stokes Bay - Gosport Angling Club

Tel: (023) 9258 4242 (Leisure Division, Gosport Borough Council)

Type:	concrete slipway
Suits:	all trailed craft
Availability:	approx. 4 hours either side HW
Restrictions:	speed limit inshore: water-skiing prohibited
Facilities:	parking for car (c) and trailer, toilets
Dues:	none
Charge:	none
Directions:	site is off roundabout at junction of Stokes Bay and Fort Roads
Waters accessed:	The Solent

Gosport (Portsmouth Harbour) - Hardway, Priory Road

Tel: (023) 9258 4242 (Leisure Division, Gosport Borough Council)

Type:	steep concrete slipway
Suits:	all craft
Availability:	approx. 4½ hours either side HW
Restrictions:	10 knot speed limit in Portsmouth Harbour: water-skiing prohibited
Facilities:	diesel, parking for car and trailer, toilets in car park, chandlery and Hardway S.C. nearby
Dues:	none
Charge:	none
Directions:	leave M27 at junction11, taking A27/A32 Gosport Rd and follow signs: site is adjacent 105 Priory Rd
Waters accessed:	Portsmouth Harbour and The Solent

Gosport (Portsmouth Harbour) - Harbour Road

Tel: (023) 9258 4242 (Leisure Division, Gosport Borough Council)

Type:	gentle but narrow concrete slipway
Suits:	small craft except pwc and windsurfers
Availability:	approx. 2½ hours either side HW
Restrictions:	10 knot speed limit in Portsmouth Harbour: water-skiing prohibited
Facilities:	fuel nearby, limited parking for car and trailer nearby, toilets, chandlery, diving supplies and outboard repairs all nearby
Dues:	none

Charge:	none
Directions:	leave M27 at jct 11 and follow signs to Gosport town centre, turning left into Harbour Road; site is on left, just before Camper and Nicholson's Boatyard
Waters accessed:	Portsmouth Harbour and The Solent

Gosport (Portsmouth Harbour) - Haslar Marina

Tel: (023) 9260 1201

Type:	shingle foreshore (1:7)
Suits:	all craft except pwc and windsurfers
Availability:	approx. 3 hours either side HW
Restrictions:	10 knot speed limit in Portsmouth Harbour: water-skiing prohibited
Facilities:	fuel nearby, parking for car and trailer, chandlery, diving supplies and outboard repairs all on site, toilets nearby
Dues:	none
Charge:	none
Directions:	leave M27 at jct 9 and follow A32 for approx. 5 miles to marina
Waters accessed:	Portsmouth Harbour and The Solent

Fareham (Portsmouth Harbour) - Lower Quay

Tel: (01329) 236100 (Fareham Borough Council)

Type:	shallow concrete ramp
Suits:	all craft up to 20'/6.1m LOA
Availability:	approx. 3 hours either side HW
Restrictions:	10 knot speed limit in Portsmouth Harbour: water-skiing prohibited; access road is narrow
Facilities:	parking for car and trailer (c), toilets and outboard repairs all nearby, chandlery on site
Dues:	none
Charge:	none
Directions:	leave M27 at junction11 and follow A27: site is adjacent Lower Quay
Waters accessed:	Portsmouth Harbour and The Solent

Paulsgrove (Portsmouth Harbour) - Southampton Road

Tel: (023) 9283 4815 (Portsmouth City Council)

Type:	concrete slipway
Suits:	small craft
Availability:	approx. 2½ hours either side HW
Restrictions:	10 knot speed limit in Portsmouth Harbour: water-skiing prohibited
Facilities:	limited parking, chandlers in Fareham
Dues:	none
Charge:	none
Directions:	leave M27 at junction11 and follow A27 east, turning off at signpost to 'Royal Navy Firefighting School'
Waters accessed:	Portsmouth Harbour and The Solent

Paulsgrove (Portsmouth Harbour) - West Bund (adjacent Port Solent)
Tel: (023) 9283 4815 (Portsmouth City Council)

Type:	concrete slipway
Suits:	all craft
Availability:	approx.1½ hours either side HW
Restrictions:	10 knot speed limit in Portsmouth Harbour: water-skiing prohibited
Facilities:	limited parking, all facilities in adjacent marina
Dues:	none
Charge:	none
Directions:	from the west, leave the M27 at junction 12; from the east, take the Hilsea exit and follow signs to Port Solent: site is 500m north of marina
Waters accessed:	Portsmouth Harbour and The Solent

Portsmouth (Portsmouth Harbour) - Port Solent Marina, South Lockside
Tel: (023) 9221 0765

Type:	launching by crane (23 ton) or boat hoist (40 ton) only
Suits:	larger craft
Availability:	0700-1700 daily by prior arrangement only
Restrictions:	10 knot speed limit in Portsmouth Harbour: water-skiing prohibited
Facilities:	fuel, parking for car and trailer, toilets, chandlery, outboard repairs, shops and restaurants all on site
Dues:	approx. £9.99
Charge:	on application
Directions:	from the west, leave the M27 at junction 12; from the east, take the Hilsea exit and follow signs to Port Solent
Waters accessed:	Portsmouth Harbour and the Solent

Portsmouth (Portsmouth Harbour) - Camber Quay, East Street
Tel: (023) 9281 4246 (Harbour Office)

Type:	wide concrete slipway
Suits:	all craft except pwc
Availability:	0800 -1600 daily by arrangement with Berthing Master
Restrictions:	10 knot speed limit in Portsmouth Harbour: pwc prohibited; locked barrier - key from Berthing Master; watch out for Isle of Wight ferries using berthing facilities opposite slipway
Facilities:	fuel nearby, parking for car and trailer, toilets and chandlery on site, other facilities available nearby
Dues:	none but licence required
Charge:	approx. £2
Directions:	follow signs to Old Portsmouth from M27/M275: site is old Isle of Wight ferry slip
Waters accessed:	Porstmouth Harbour and the Solent

Eastney (Langstone Harbour) - Eastney Beach
Tel: (023) 9246 3419 (Harbour Office)

Type:	concrete slipway often covered by sand and shingle
Suits:	all craft: beware strong tidal currents, especially on spring tides
Availability:	all states of tide
Restrictions:	10 knot speed limit in Langstone Harbour: water-skiing permitted in designated area under licence only; pwc require a transit permit; Langstone Harbour is an area of international importance for nature conservation: landing in many areas is prohibited, especially from May to November
Facilities:	parking for car and trailer and toilets nearby
Dues:	no additional fee
Charge:	approx.£6.50 daily (£25.75 p.a.): pwc £17.30 daily (£64.90 p.a.)
Directions:	from M27/A27 follow A2030 and signs to Southsea, turning off to follow signs to Langstone Marina and Fort Cumberland: site is just south of Eastney C.A. clubhouse
Waters accessed:	Langstone Harbour and the Solent

Havant (Langstone Harbour) - Brockhampton Quay
Tel: (023) 9246 3419 (Harbour Office)

Type:	wide concrete slipway
Suits:	all craft
Availability:	approx. 1½ hours either side HW
Restrictions:	10 knot speed limit in Langstone Harbour: water-skiing permitted in designated area only under licence; pwc require transit permit through harbour; access has height restriction; Langstone Harbour is an area of international importance for nature conservation: landing in many areas is prohibited, especially from May to November
Facilities:	parking for car and trailer on site
Dues:	no additional fee
Charge:	approx. £6.50 daily (£25.75 pa) : pwc £17.30 daily (£64.90 pa)
Directions:	fom A27 follow signs to the Public Amenity Tip and Broadmarsh
Waters accessed:	Langstone Harbour and the Solent

Hayling Island (Langstone Harbour) - Ferry Point
Tel: (023) 9246 3419 (Harbour Office)

Type:	wide concrete slipway
Suits:	all craft: trailer-sailers must be rigged clear of the slip and turning area
Availability:	all states of tide, but seek advice at or near LW or if over 25'/7.6m LOA

Restrictions:	10 knot speed limit in Langstone Harbour: water-skiing permitted in designated area under licence only; pwc require transit permit through harbour; divers require permission; Langstone Harbour is an area of international importance for nature conservation: landing in many areas is prohibited, especially from May to November
Facilities:	fuel, parking for car nearby and for trailer on site (c), toilets on site, pub adjacent
Dues:	no additional fee
Charge:	approx. £6.50 daily (£25.75 pa): pwc £17.30 daily (£64.90 pa)
Directions:	from A27 follow signs to Hayling Is, going to seafront and then turning right and following road to end; site is on western tip of island and adjacent Harbour Office and Ferry Boat Inn
Waters accessed:	Langstone Harbour and The Solent

Hayling Island (Chichester Harbour) - Hayling Yacht Co Ltd

Tel: (023) 9246 3592

Type:	concrete slipway (1:8)
Suits:	all craft except pwc
Availability:	approx. 2 hours before HW to 2½ hours after during daylight hours: phone to make sure slipway is unobstructed
Restrictions:	8 knot speed limit in Chichester Harbour: water-skiing and pwc prohibited; Harbour Office and Patrol (Apr-Oct) listen on VHF Ch 14
Facilities:	diesel on site, petrol nearby, parking for car and trailer, toilets, chandlery and full boatyard facilities all on site
Dues:	approx. £3
Charge:	approx. £6
Directions:	follow signs to Hayling Is from A27, crossing bridge and following main road for 2 miles; pass two pubs and entrance is 300m on left; access is via Mill Rythe Lane
Waters accessed:	Chichester Harbour and the Solent

Hayling Island (Chichester Harbour) - Northney Marina, Northney Road

Tel: (023) 9246 6321

Type:	concrete slipway into marina
Suits:	all craft especially trailer-sailers: no pwc
Availability:	all states of tide
Restrictions:	8 knot speed limit in Chichester Harbour: water-skiing and pwc prohibited
Facilities:	diesel and LPG on site, petrol nearby, parking for car and trailer on site, toilets, chandlery, outboard repairs and all yard facilities, bar and restaurant all available on site; Harbour Office and Patrol (Apr-Oct) listen on VHF Ch 14
Dues:	approx. £3
Charge:	approx. £13

Directions: from M27/A27 turn off to Hayling Is turning left immediately after crossing bridge into Northney Road and turning left into marina

Waters accessed: Chichester and Langstone Harbours and the Solent

Hayling Island (Chichester Harbour) - Shore Watersports, Northney

Tel: (023) 9246 7334

Type:	concrete slipway
Suits:	sailing dinghies and windsurfers: no pwc
Availability:	approx. 2-3 hours either side HW
Restrictions:	8 knot speed limit in Chichester Harbour: water-skiing and pwc prohibited; this is a very popular site for windsurfers
Facilities:	diesel and LPG on site, petrol nearby, parking for car and trailer on site, toilets, chandlery, outboard repairs and all yard facilities, bar and restaurant all available in marina; windsurfing shop; Harbour Office and Patrol (Apr-Oct) listen on VHF Ch 14
Dues:	approx. £3
Charge:	none
Directions:	from M27/A27 turn off to Hayling Is turning left immediately after crossing bridge into Northney Road and turning into marina entrance; site is on left
Waters accessed:	Chichester and Langstone Harbours and the Solent

Langstone (Chichester Harbour) - Ship Inn

Tel: (01243) 512301 (Harbour Office, Itchenor)

Type:	concrete slipway
Suits:	small craft only: no pwc
Availability:	approx. 2 hours either side HW
Restrictions:	8 knot speed limit in Chichester Harbour: water-skiing and pwc prohibited
Facilities:	fuel from garage over bridge, parking for car and trailer, toilets in pub; Harbour Office and Patrol (Apr-Oct) listen on VHF Ch 14
Dues:	approx. £3
Charge:	no separate fee
Directions:	from M27/A27 turn off onto A3023 to Hayling Is turning left immediately before bridge: site is adjacent to the 'Ship Inn'
Waters accessed:	Chichester Harbour, Langstone Harbour and The Solent

Emsworth (Chichester Harbour) - Warblington Road

Tel: (01243) 376422 (Harbour Office, Emsworth)

Type:	shingle hard
Suits:	small craft only: no pwc
Availability:	approx. 2 hours either side HW
Restrictions:	8 knot speed limit in Chichester Harbour: water-skiing and pwc prohibited

Facilities:	limited parking and turning in road, toilets, chandlery and all other facilities nearby; Harbour Office and Patrol (Apr-Oct) listen on VHF Ch 14
Dues:	approx. £3
Charge:	no additional fee
Directions:	from A27 Portsmouth-Chichester road turn off just west of Emsworth into Warblington Rd: site is at end of road
Waters accessed:	Chichester Harbour and The Solent

Emsworth (Chichester Harbour) - South Street

Tel: (01243) 376422 (Harbour Office, Emsworth)

Type:	concrete slipway onto shingle
Suits:	all craft except pwc
Availability:	approx. 3 hours either side HW
Restrictions:	8 knot speed limit in Chichester Harbour: water-skiing and pwc prohibited; Harbour Office and Patrol (Apr-Oct) listen on VHF Ch 14
Facilities:	parking and toilets in car park at top of street, chandlers opposite, other facilities nearby
Dues:	approx. £3
Charge:	approx. £1.70
Directions:	from A27 Portsmouth-Chichester road turn off into Emsworth
Waters accessed:	Chichester Harbour and the Solent

Emsworth (Chichester Harbour) - Emsworth Yacht Harbour Ltd

Tel: (01243) 375211

Type:	concrete ramp
Suits:	all craft except pwc
Availability:	approx. 2½ hours either side HW by prior arrangement
Restrictions:	8 knot speed limit in Chichester Harbour: water-skiing and pwc prohibited; Harbour Office and Patrol (Apr-Oct) listen on VHF Ch 14
Facilities:	petrol nearby, diesel, parking for car and trailer (c), toilets and showers, outboard repairs and chandlery all on site
Dues:	approx. £3
Charge:	approx. £6
Directions:	from A27 Portsmouth-Chichester road turn off east of Emsworth and follow signs: site is at the north end of Thorney Is and access is via Thorney Road
Waters accessed:	Chichester Harbour and the Solent

Prinsted (Chichester Harbour)

Tel: (01243) 512301 (Harbour Office, Itchenor)

Type:	shingle hard
Suits:	small craft only: no pwc
Availability:	approx. 2 hours either side HW

Restrictions:	8 knot speed limit in Chichester Harbour: water-skiing and pwc prohibited; Harbour Office and Patrol (Apr-Oct) listen on VHF Ch 14
Facilities:	limited parking for car and trailer, chandlery in Emsworth
Dues:	approx. £3
Charge:	no additional fee
Directions:	from A27 Portsmouth-Chichester road turn off east of Emsworth following signs: site is at end of road south of the village
Waters accessed:	Chichester Harbour and the Solent

Bosham (Chichester Harbour) - Bosham Lane

Tel: (01243) 512301 (Harbour Office, Itchenor)

Type:	shingle hard
Suits:	small craft only: no pwc
Availability:	approx. 3 hours either side HW
Restrictions:	8 knot speed limit in Chichester Harbour: water-skiing and pwc prohibited
Facilities:	parking for car and trailer (c) and toilets in car park nearby; Harbour Office and Patrol (Apr-Oct) listen on VHF Ch 14
Dues:	approx. £3
Charge:	no additional fee
Directions:	from Chichester follow A27, turning onto A259 and following signs: site is at the end of Bosham Lane
Waters accessed:	Chichester Harbour and the Solent

Bosham (Chichester Harbour) - The Quay

Tel: (01243) 573336 (Quaymaster)

Type:	concrete slipway onto shingle and mud
Suits:	small craft only: no pwc
Availability:	at all states of tide
Restrictions:	8 knot speed limit in Chichester Harbour: water-skiing and pwc prohibited
Facilities:	no parking on quay but parking for car and trailer (c) and toilets in car park in Bosham Lane; crane; Harbour Office and patrol (Apr-Oct) listen on VHF Ch 14
Dues:	approx. £3
Charge:	on application
Directions:	from Chichester follow A27, turning onto A259 and following signs: site is on the Quay and access is often congested
Waters accessed:	Chichester Harbour and The Solent

Dell Quay (Chichester Harbour)

Tel: (01243) 512301 (Harbour Office, Itchenor)

Type:	shingle hard
Suits:	small craft only: no pwc
Availability:	approx. 2½ hours either side HW

Restrictions:	8 knot speed limit in Chichester Harbour: water-skiing and pwc prohibited
Facilities:	limited parking for car and trailer, pub; Harbour Office and Patrol (Apr-Oct) listen on VHF Ch 14
Dues:	approx. £3
Charge:	no additional fee
Directions:	from Chichester follow A27, turning onto A286 and following signs: site is at the end of road adjacent to Quay
Waters accessed:	Chichester Harbour and The Solent

Birdham (Chichester Harbour) - Chichester Marina

Tel: (01243) 512731

Type:	shallow concrete ramp into locked marina basin
Suits:	powered craft with less than 4'/1.2m draught and up to 25'/7.6m LOA
Availability:	approx. 5 hours either side HW; contact basin office or lock control on arrival
Restrictions:	8 knot speed limit in Chichester Harbour: water-skiing and pwc prohibited; Harbour Office and Patrol (Apr-Oct) listen on VHF Ch 14; access code to locked barrier issued on payment of fee
Facilities:	fuel, parking for car and trailer, toilets, chandlery, yard facilities, bar all available on site; outboard repairs from Itchenor
Dues:	approx. £3
Charge:	approx. £14.69
Directions:	take the A286 off the A27 Chichester by-pass signposted to E/W Wittering, turning right to marina after 2 miles
Waters accessed:	Chichester Harbour and the Solent

Itchenor (Chichester Harbour)

Tel: (01243) 512301 (Harbour Office)

Type:	large shingle hard
Suits:	all craft except pwc
Availability:	all states of tide
Restrictions:	8 knot speed limit in Chichester Harbour: water-skiing and pwc prohibited; no parking on hard
Facilities:	parking for car and trailer in car park (c), toilets, outboard repairs, pub, boatyards; Harbour Office and Patrol (Apr-Oct) listen on VHF Ch 14
Dues:	approx. £3: pay Warden on site
Charge:	approx. £1.70: pay Warden on site
Directions:	take the A286 off the A27 Chichester by-pass to E/W Wittering, turning off to Itchenor after 8 miles: site is at end of road
Waters accessed:	Chichester Harbour and the Solent

Bracklesham
Tel: (01243) 534799 (Leisure and Tourism Dept. Chichester D.C.)

Type: concrete slipway onto shingle beach
Suits: all craft except pwc
Availability: all states of tide
Restrictions: 8 knot speed limit within 300m MLWS mark with buoyed access channel; pwc prohibited; vehicles other than licensed tractors not permitted on beach
Facilities: fuel nearby, parking for car and trailer (c), toilets and cafe on site
Dues: none
Charge: none
Directions: take the A286 off the A27 Chichester by-pass signposted to E/W Wittering, turning onto B2198: turn left at end of road into E Bracklesham Drive and access is through car park
Waters accessed: Bracklesham Bay and the Solent

Selsey - East Beach Amenity Ramp
Tel: (01243) 534799 (Leisure and Tourism Dept. Chichester D.C.)

Type: wooden ramp onto shingle beach may be covered with shingle
Suits: small craft which can be manhandled only: no pwc
Availability: approx. 2-3 hours either side HW or at all times over the beach
Restrictions: 8 knot speed limit within 300m MLWS mark with buoyed access channel: pwc prohibited; there are strong currents in this area and this site is not suitable for launching in onshore winds
Facilities: fuel from garage, parking for car and trailer (c), toilets and cafe all on site
Dues: none
Charge: none
Directions: from Chichester or A27 take B2145 and B2201: site is signposted from main street and access is through large car park
Waters accessed: English Channel

Bognor Regis - Gloucester Road
Tel: (01903) 716133 ext. 3321 (Arun D.C.)

Type: wide concrete ramp with wooden sides onto sand
Suits: small powered craft and pwc
Availability: all states of tide
Restrictions: 8 knot speed limit in buoyed area within 300m of MLW mark: water-skiing and pwc permitted outside this area; may be locked height barrier
Facilities: fuel from garage (not sun), limited parking for car and trailer (c), toilets nearby
Dues: none

Charge:	approx. £8
Directions:	from Chichester follow A27 east turning onto A259 and B2166 and follow signs to seafront: access is through car park at east end
Waters accessed:	English Channel

Littlehampton (River Arun) - Littlehampton Marina, Ferry Road
Tel: (01903) 713553

Type:	wide shallow concrete ramp
Suits:	powered craft except pwc
Availability:	approx. 4 hours either side HW by prior arrangement 0800 - 1700
Restrictions:	6½ knot speed limit in river: windsurfing, water-skiing and pwc prohibited, launching by yard staff only and insurance certificate required for craft; tides run very strongly in river entrance
Facilities:	fuel, parking for car and trailer, toilets and showers, crane and hoist (for craft up to 45 tons), chandlery, dive shop, outboard repairs and full boatyard facilities; site for tents/camper vans
Dues:	approx. £5
Charge:	approx. £18.80 (mon-fri), £23.50 (sat, sun & BH)
Directions:	from Chichester follow A27 east to Arundel, taking the A284 then A259; cross river and turn left after ½ mile: site is on west bank downstream of bridge and approx. 1 mile from the sea
Waters accessed:	River Arun (navigable for 24 miles inland) and open sea

Ford (River Arun) - Ship and Anchor Marina
Tel: (01243) 551262

Type:	concrete slipway
Suits:	powered craft up to 24'/7.3m LOA: no pwc
Availability:	approx. 4 hours either side HW 0900 - 1730
Restrictions:	6½ knot speed limit in river: launching by yard staff only using tractor at owner's risk; proof of insurance required; tides in river entrance run strongly
Facilities:	parking for car and trailer, toilets, campsite and pub
Dues:	none
Charge:	approx. £25
Directions:	from the A27 at Arundel take the Ford road: site is on left after the station
Waters accessed:	River Arun (navigable for 24 miles inland) and open sea

Pulborough (River Arun) - Old Swan Bridge, Swan Corner

Type:	steep concrete slipway with turning space and snatch blocks at top
Suits:	canoes and small powered craft up to 15'/4.6m LOA: no pwc
Availability:	near HW only

Restrictions:	5½ knot speed limit in river (6½ knots below Arundel Bridge): access is narrow and difficult; a min. 40m of rope is required to lower boat
Facilities:	fuel nearby, parking at station nearby (c), toilets nearby, pub
Dues:	none
Charge:	none
Directions:	turn off the A29 Bognor road at junction with A283: site is adjacent east side of bridge on north bank
Waters accessed:	River Arun (navigable for 24 miles inland) and open sea

Littlehampton (River Arun) - Fisherman's Quay, Surrey Street
Tel: (01903) 721215 (Harbour Office)

Type:	steep concrete slipway(1:7) with sharp lip at summit onto mud
Suits:	all craft except pwc
Availability:	all states of tide but concrete only extends to half tide mark and thereafter is compacted mud: beware strong currents in river entrance especially at springs
Restrictions:	6½ knot speed limit in harbour and river: water-skiing, windsurfing and pwc prohibited in harbour and river
Facilities:	fuel nearby, parking for car and trailer under 14'/4.3m long on site (c), chandlery, diving supplies and outboard repairs adjacent
Dues:	approx. £5
Charge:	no additional fee charged
Directions:	follow A284 from Arundel and signs to town centre: site is at end of Surrey St on east bank of river adjacent to Lifeboat Station
Waters accessed:	River Arun (navigable for 24 miles inland) and open sea

Worthing - Sea Place Car Park, Marine Crescent
Tel: (01903) 238977 (Foreshore Manager, Worthing B.C.)

Type:	shallow wooden ramp onto shingle beach
Suits:	small craft which can be manhandled
Availability:	approx. 3 hours either side HW
Restrictions:	8 knot speed limit within buoyed area: slipway has locked barrier and access has height restriction of 4'6"/1.3m; car park is very congested in summer; no vehicles allowed on Promenade
Facilities:	fuel nearby, parking for car and trailer on site (c), toilets nearby
Dues:	none
Charge:	none
Directions:	follow seafront road approx. 2½ miles west from town centre
Waters accessed:	English Channel

Worthing - Alinora Car Park, Marine Crescent

Tel: (01903) 238977 (Foreshore Manager, Worthing B.C.)

Type:	shallow wooden ramp onto shingle beach
Suits:	small craft which can be manhandled only
Availability:	approx. 3 hours either side HW
Restrictions:	8 knot speed limit within buoyed area: slipway has locked barrier and access is through car park with 5'/1.5m height restriction which can be very congested in summer; no vehicles allowed on Promenade
Facilities:	fuel nearby, parking for car and trailer on site (c), toilets nearby
Dues:	none
Charge:	none
Directions:	follow seafront road west for approx. 3 miles from town centre
Waters accessed:	English Channel

Shoreham Beach - Emerald Quay

Tel: (01273) 598100 (Port Office)

Type:	concrete slipway
Suits:	dinghies and small powerboats
Availability:	approx. 2 hours either side HW
Restrictions:	10 mph speed limit in harbour: water-skiing permitted in designated area in river; pwc and windsurfing prohibited
Facilities:	fuel nearby, limited parking for car and trailer adjacent or in car park (c) nearby
Dues:	approx. £3.30 per month or £16.90 p.a.
Charge:	no separate fee
Directions:	turn off A259 after crossing Norfolk Bridge and follow signs to Shoreham Beach: site is off Riverside Road just before Emerald Quay Housing Estate
Waters accessed:	River Adur, Shoreham Harbour and English Channel

Shoreham (River Adur) - Ropetackle, Little High Street Hard

Tel: (01273) 598100 (Port Office)

Type:	tarmac road onto shingle and mud
Suits:	dinghies and small powerboats
Availability:	approx. 2-3 hours either side HW
Restrictions:	10 mph speed limit: water-skiing permitted in designated area upstream but not in port waters; pwc and wind-surfing prohibited
Facilities:	fuel, parking for car and trailer (c), chandlers and boatyard nearby
Dues:	approx. £3.30 per month; £16.90 p.a.
Charge:	no separate fee
Directions:	from A24 take A283 to Shoreham turning right after Ballamys' Garage into Little High St: site is upstream of the Norfolk Bridge
Waters accessed:	River Adur, Shoreham Harbour and English Channel

Shoreham Harbour - Lady Bee Marina, Albion Street
Tel: (0273) 593801

Type:	short and shallow concrete and steel slipway into locked harbour
Suits:	all craft up to 26'/7.9m LOA and 3'/1m draught except pwc
Availability:	0830-1800 mon-sat, 1000-1400 sun but subject to lock gates opening 4 hours either side HW
Restrictions:	4 knot speed limit in harbour, water-skiing and pwc prohibited; telephone to check availability
Facilities:	fuel nearby, limited parking, toilets, and showers, chandlery
Dues:	none
Charge:	approx. £16.50 for launch, recovery and use of lock
Directions:	turn off main coast road between Brighton and Worthing (A259) opposite Shoreham Harbour entrance into Albion St
Waters accessed:	Shoreham Harbour, River Adur and English Channel

Newhaven - Newhaven Marina, Fort Road
Tel: (01273) 513881

Type:	two steep concrete slipways in marina (1) at Russell Simpson Marine (01273) 612612 (2) at Andy Pace Marine (01273 516010)
Suits:	craft up to 20'/6.1m LOA: no pwc
Availability:	2½ hours either side HW from 0900 -1800: phone to check for availability
Restrictions:	5 knot speed limit in harbour: pwc prohibited
Facilities:	diesel on site, petrol nearby, parking for car and trailer on site, toilets and showers, chandlery, cafe, outboard repairs, diving supplies, yacht club all on site
Dues:	no separate charge
Charge:	approx. £12.50; season ticket available
Directions:	follow M23/A23 to Brighton, then A259 coast road 7 miles to Newhaven: turn off one-way system to follow signs to Newhaven Fort, then turn left opposite the Sheffield Arms and site is 100m on right; site is on west bank of river
Waters accessed:	River Ouse and English Channel

Eastbourne - Sovereign Harbour
Tel: (01323) 470099

Type:	50 ton boat hoist
Suits:	trailer-sailers and larger craft
Availability:	by prior arrangement
Restrictions:	5 knot speed limit in harbour and channel: two access barriers with phones to Harbour Office; twin locks are manned 24hrs a day; boats launched must have 3rd party insurance for £1m

Facilities:	fuel, parking for car and trailer, toilets and showers, chandlery, LPG, pumpout, outboard repairs, shops and restaurants
Dues:	no separate fee
Charge:	£27.50 daily 0830-1000 and 1530-1700 1st May to 30th Sept: £35 launch/recovery and night afloat at weekends
Directions:	follow seafront east from Eastbourne town centre towards Pevensey Bay following signs to Sovereign Harbour
Waters accessed:	English Channel

Bexhill-on-Sea - West Parade
Tel: (01424) 787878 (Beach Inspector, Rother D.C.)

Type:	concrete slipway onto shingle beach
Suits:	small craft which can be manhandled
Availability:	approx. 3 hours either side HW
Restrictions:	8 knot speed limit within 100m of shore: designated lanes give access for water-skiing; vehicles are not allowed on the promenade so craft must be pushed
Facilities:	fuel (1/2 mile), parking for car and trailer on site, toilets and cafe nearby
Dues:	none
Charge:	none
Directions:	follow signs to seafront from A259
Waters accessed:	English Channel

Rye Harbour (River Rother) - Rye Harbour Village
Tel: (01797) 225225 Fax: (01797) 227429 (Harbour Master)

Type:	concrete slipway
Suits:	all craft except windsurfers
Availability:	approx. 2 hours before HW to 3 hours after
Restrictions:	6 knot speed limit in river is robustly enforced: pwc are restricted and water-skiing permitted in river for club members only; narrow harbour entrance with bar and strong tidal flow: vessels must not enter or leave harbour against the direction of the Harbour Master
Facilities:	fuel nearby, parking for car and trailer on site, toilets, chandlery, pub, sailing club, shop, yard facilities and ouboard repairs nearby; call Hbr Mr for information on weather, tides etc.
Dues:	approx. £10 per day, £85 p.a.
Charge:	no additional fee charged
Directions:	follow A259 to Rye and then signs to Rye Harbour
Waters accessed:	River Rother and the English Channel

New Romney - Varne Boat Club, The Greens, Littlestone

Tel: (01797) 362993 (Clubhouse) or (01797) 367597 (Membership Sec.)

Type:	assisted launching from shallow concrete ramp
Suits:	all craft up to 25'/7.6m LOA
Availability:	approx. 3 hours either side HW by prior arrangement
Restrictions:	5 knot speed limit inside marker buoys: water-skiing permitted in designated area
Facilities:	fuel nearby, parking for car and trailer, toilets and showers, changing rooms and refreshments all on site
Dues:	none
Charge:	approx. £16 with assistance
Directions:	follow A259 to New Romney turning right onto the B2071 to Littlestone; club is on foreshore on left next to RNLI station
Waters accessed:	Romney Bay and the English Channel

Folkestone - Inner Harbour Slipway

Tel: (01303) 715305 (Port Office)

Type:	medium concrete slipway
Suits:	all craft
Availability:	approx. 2-3 hours either side HW: report to small cafe adjacent to site to pay fees
Restrictions:	5 mph speed limit in Inner Harbour: access to site restricted by narrow and low arches
Facilities:	fuel, parking for car and trailer, toilets, chandlery, diving supplies, outboard repairs and other facilities all available nearby
Dues:	approx. £2.50
Charge:	no additional fee charged
Directions:	from M20/A20 follow signs to Folkestone Harbour
Waters accessed:	Folkestone Harbour and the English Channel

Dover - The Promenade

Tel: (01304) 241663 (Berthing Master)

Type:	shallow concrete ramp into Outer Harbour
Suits:	small craft up to 12'/3.6m LOA which can be manhandled: no pwc
Availability:	at all times
Restrictions:	8 knot speed limit in harbour: due to constant shipping movements, craft are not allowed to enter east of the reclaim or go to northern edge of anchorage; craft wishing to leave harbour must contact Port Control on VHF Ch 74 or 16 call sign 'Dover Port Control'
Facilities:	fuel nearby, parking for car nearby (but not on Promenade) and for trailer on site (c), toilets, chandlery, outboard repairs nearby
Dues:	none
Charge:	none

Directions:	follow A2 to Eastern Docks, then along Marine Parade: site is opposite Royal Cinque Ports Y.C. and access is via Promenade
Waters accessed:	Dover Harbour and the English Channel

Dover - Dover Marina, Wellington Dock

Tel: (01304) 241663

Type:	launching by 50 ton boat hoist into locked basin
Suits:	larger craft
Availability:	0800-1600 daily
Restrictions:	8 knot speed limit in harbour: due to constant shipping movements, craft are not allowed to enter east of the reclaim or go to northern edge of anchorage; craft wishing to leave harbour must contact Port Control on VHF Ch 74 or 16 call sign 'Dover Port Control'
Facilities:	fuel, parking for car and trailer (by permit only c), toilets and showers, all marina facilities, Royal Cinque Ports Y.C. nearby
Dues:	none
Charge:	on application
Directions:	follow signs from M20/A20
Waters accessed:	Dover Harbour and English Channel

St Margaret's-at-Cliffe

Tel: (01304) 821199 (Recreation Officer, Dover D.C.)

Type:	shallow concrete ramp onto beach may be covered by shingle
Suits:	all craft
Availability:	all states of tide but best at HW
Restrictions:	10 mph speed limit within 150m of LW mark with access lane; water-skiing is permitted offshore; access to site is via steep narrow road
Facilities:	fuel nearby, parking for car and trailer (c), toilets, refreshments all on site
Dues:	none
Charge:	none
Directions:	from Dover follow A2 to top of Jubilee Way turning onto A258 to Deal; turn right onto B2058 to St Margaret's and follow signs to St Margaret's Bay
Waters accessed:	St Margaret's Bay and English Channel

Deal - Kingsdown Slipway

Tel: (01304) 821199 (Recreation Officer, Dover D.C.)

Type:	two wooden ramps onto shingle
Suits:	small craft up to 17'/5.2m LOA
Availability:	all states of tide but best at HW
Restrictions:	10 mph speed limit within 150m of LW mark with access channels for water-skiing: access to 2nd slip-way is through locked barrier
Facilities:	fuel, parking for car and trailer, toilets, pub
Dues:	none

Charge:	none
Directions:	from A258 to Deal follow signs (for large vehicles) to Kingsdown, then Walmer and turn into Kingsdown Road
Waters accessed:	Dover Strait and English Channel

Deal - North End Ramps

Tel: (01304) 821199 (Recreation Officer, Dover D.C.)

Type:	two steep concrete ramps onto shingle foreshore
Suits:	small craft which can be manhandled
Availability:	all states of tide, Apr - Oct
Restrictions:	access to site closed Oct - Apr due to risk of flooding; no cars allowed on Promenade
Facilities:	fuel nearby, limited parking for car and trailer and other facilities nearby
Dues:	none
Charge:	none
Directions:	from Dover follow A2 to top of Jubilee Way turning onto A258 to Deal: site is accessed from the Promenade
Waters accessed:	Dover Strait and English Channel

Sandwich (River Stour) - Town Quay

Tel: (01304) 821199 (Recreation Officer, Dover D.C.)

Type:	steep concrete ramp
Suits:	all craft up to 20'/6.1m LOA
Availability:	approx. 2 hours either side HW
Restrictions:	6 and 8 knot speed limits in river
Facilities:	fuel from local garage, parking for car and trailer and toilets on site, chandlery and boatyard facilities nearby
Dues:	none
Charge:	none
Directions:	from Canterbury follow A256 east then signs to town centre
Waters accessed:	River Stour and Pegwell Bay

Ramsgate - Harbour Slipway, Military Road

Tel: (01843) 592277 (Harbour Master)

Type:	granite block slipway into locked Inner Harbour
Suits:	larger craft: no pwc
Availability:	at all times but lock gates only open 2 hours either side of HW
Restrictions:	5 knot speed limit in harbour: locked gate at top of slipway; Harbour Master's permission must be obtained in advance
Facilities:	fuel, parking for car and trailer (c), toilets, tractor and crane available, launderette, cafe, chandlers nearby
Dues:	no additional charge
Charge:	approx. £40 + vat

Directions:	from Canterbury follow A28/A253 to Ramsgate and signs to ferry terminal: site is in Military Road
Waters accessed:	English Channel

Ramsgate - Eastcliff, Marina Esplanade
Tel: (01843) 577529 (Thanet Distrcit Council)

Type:	concrete ramp
Suits:	pwc only
Availability:	approx. 2 hours either side HW
Restrictions:	launching for pwc only: membership of T.D.C. Water Safety Group required - contact number above for details
Facilities:	fuel nearby, parking for car and trailer on site (c), other facilities nearby
Dues:	none
Charge:	none
Directions:	follow the Madeira Walk road up from Ramsgate Harbour to the Eastern Esplanade and take the first right down to the beach
Waters accessed:	English Channel

Broadstairs - Harbour Slipway
Tel: (01843) 861879 Harbour Master

Type:	wooden slipway
Suits:	small craft which can be manhandled only
Availability:	at HW only
Restrictions:	5 knot speed limit in harbour: no vehicle access to slipway
Facilities:	fuel from garage (1/2 mile), parking for car and trailer, toilets
Dues:	not known
Charge:	yes
Directions:	from Margate or Ramsgate follow A255
Waters accessed:	English Channel

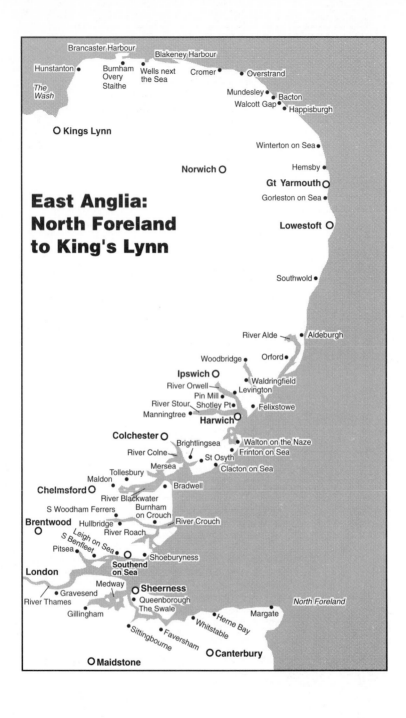

Brancaster Harbour
Blakeney Harbour
Hunstanton ●
Burnham Overy Staithe ●
Wells next the Sea
Cromer ●
Overstrand ●
Mundesley ● ● Bacton
Walcott Gap ● ● Happisburgh
The Wash

O **Kings Lynn**

Winterton on Sea ●
Norwich O
Hemsby ●
Gt Yarmouth O
Gorleston on Sea ●

East Anglia: North Foreland to King's Lynn

Lowestoft O

Southwold ●

River Alde ─── ● Aldeburgh

Woodbridge ● Orford ●
Ipswich O
River Orwell ─ ● Waldringfield
Pin Mill ● Levington
River Stour ─ Shotley Pt ● ● Felixstowe
Manningtree ● **Harwich** O

Colchester O
Brightlingsea ● ● Walton on the Naze
River Colne ─ ● Frinton on Sea
Mersea ● St Osyth
Tollesbury ● Clacton on Sea
Maldon ●
Chelmsford O ● Bradwell
River Blackwater
S Woodham Ferrers Burnham on Crouch
Brentwood O Hullbridge ● ● River Crouch
Leigh on Sea River Roach
S Benfleet
Pitsea ● ● Shoeburyness
London **Southend on Sea** O
Medway O **Sheerness**
● Gravesend Queenborough
River Thames The Swale
Gillingham ● North Foreland
Margate
● Herne Bay
Sittingbourne ● Whitstable
● Faversham
O **Canterbury**
O **Maidstone**

Margate - Foreness Bay, Cliftonville

Tel: (01843) 577529 (Foreshore Office, Thanet District Council)

Type:	concrete slipway onto beach
Suits:	powered craft except pwc
Availability:	approx. 2 hours either side HW
Restrictions:	8 knot speed limit within 400m of shore: this is a designated water-skiing area operated by Foreness Ski Club; sailing craft are prohibited; access permitted only to members of T.D.C. Water Safety Group - contact number above for details
Facilities:	fuel from garage (1 mile), parking for car and trailer, toilets
Dues:	none
Charge:	none
Directions:	from Canterbury follow A 28 to Cliftonville seafront, E of Margate
Waters accessed:	Thames Estuary

Margate - Palm Bay, Cliftonville

Tel: (01843) 577529 (Foreshore Office, Thanet District Council)

Type:	launching over sand
Suits:	pwc only
Availability:	approx. 2 hours either side HW
Restrictions:	site is for use of pwc only - no other activities permitted: access only to members of T.D.C. Water Safety Group - contact number above for details
Facilities:	fuel nearby, parking for car and trailer, toilets and showers, cafe on site
Dues:	none
Charge:	approx. £10
Directions:	from Canterbury, follow A28 to Cliftonville seafront on east side of Margate town centre; access is via Princes Walk
Waters accessed:	Thames Estuary

Margate - Harbour Slip

Tel: (01843) 861879 (Broadstairs Harbour Master)

Type:	concrete ramp onto sand
Suits:	all craft except pwc and windsurfers
Availability:	approx. 2 hours either side HW
Restrictions:	8 knot speed limit within 400m HW mark: water-skiing permitted in designated area; contact Hb Mr or join T.D.C. Water Safety Group Tel: (01843) 577529 Foreshore Officer, Thanet District Council
Facilities:	fuel nearby, parking for car and trailer (c) and toilets on site, chandlery, diving supplies and repairs available nearby; Margate Y.C, adjacent
Dues:	yes
Charge:	yes
Directions:	from Canterbury follow A28 to town centre and signs to harbour
Waters accessed:	Thames Estuary

Margate - Westbrook Bay, Royal Esplanade

Tel: (01843) 577529 (Foreshore Officer, Thanet D.C.)

Type:	concrete ramp onto firm sand
Suits:	small powered craft: no pwc or windsurfers
Availability:	approx. 2 hours either side HW
Restrictions:	8 knot speed limit within 400m shore: this is a designated water-skiing area and other activities are not permitted; to gain access you need to be a member of the T.D.C. Water Safety Group - contact number above for details
Facilities:	fuel nearby, parking for car and trailer on site (c), toilets and other facilities available nearby
Dues:	none
Charge:	none
Directions:	from Canterbury follow A28 to Margate and take coast road west
Waters accessed:	Thames Estuary

Margate - Winter Gardens, Fort Promenade

Tel: (01843) 577529 (Foreshore Officer, Thanet D.C.)

Type:	concrete ramp
Suits:	pwc only
Availability:	approx. 2 hours either side HW
Restrictions:	access only to members of T.D.C. Water Safety Group - contact number above for details
Facilities:	fuel nearby, parking for car and trailer (c), toilets, chandlery and outboard repairs on site,diving supplies nearby
Dues:	none
Charge:	none
Directions:	from Canterbury follow A28 to town centre and signs to harbour, then turn left onto Fort Promenade
Waters accessed:	Thames Estuary

Margate - St Mildreds, Westgate Esplanade

Tel: (01843) 577529 (Foreshore Officer, Thanet D.C.)

Type:	concrete slipway onto firm sand
Suits:	sailing dinghies, trailer-sailers and small powered craft
Availability:	approx. 2 hours either side HW
Restrictions:	8 knot speed limit within 400m shore: speed boats & pwc prohibited; no launching between 0900-1800 June to Sept; available only to members of the T.D.C.Water Safety Group - contact number above for details; no vehicles permitted on beach
Facilities:	fuel nearby, parking for car and trailer (c), toilets and cafe on site, chandlery, diving supplies and outboard repairs available nearby
Dues:	none
Charge:	none
Directions:	from Margate follow A28 towards Canterbury: turn right into Westbrook Ave then right again into St Mildreds Ave
Waters accessed:	Thames Estuary

Margate - West Bay, Westgate, West Ramp
Tel: (01843) 577529 (Foreshore Officer, Thanet D.C.)

Type:	concrete ramp
Suits:	sailing and small powered craft: no speed boats or pwc
Availability:	approx. 2 hours either side HW
Restrictions:	8 knot speed limit within 400m shore: to gain access join the T.D.C.Water Safety Group - contact number above for details
Facilities:	fuel nearby, parking for car and trailer, toilets and cafe on site, other facilities available nearby
Dues:	none
Charge:	none
Directions:	from Margate follow A28 towards Canterbury: turn right into Westbrook Ave and at end of road turn right onto West Bay
Waters accessed:	Thames Estuary

Margate - West Bay, Westgate, East Ramp
Tel: (01843) 577529 (Foreshore Officer, Thanet D.C.)

Type:	concrete slipway onto firm sand
Suits:	sailing dinghies, trailer-sailers up to 14'/4.3m LOA and small powered craft: no pwc or ski-boats
Availability:	approx. 2 hours either side HW
Restrictions:	8 knot speed limit within 400m of shore: pwc, wind-surfing and water-skiing prohibited; to gain access you must join the T.D.C. Water Safety Group - contact the number above for details; hand-launching only permitted from June-Sept
Facilities:	fuel nearby, parking for car and trailer (c), toilets and cafe on site, other facilities nearby
Dues:	none
Charge:	none
Directions:	from Margate follow A28 towards Canterbury: turn right into Westbrook Ave and at end of road turn right onto West Bay
Waters accessed:	Thames Estuary

Margate - Beresford Gap, Beach Avenue, Birchington
Tel: (01843) 577529 (Foreshore Officer, Thanet D.C.)

Type:	steep concrete slipway onto Promenade
Suits:	ski-boats only
Availability:	approx. 2 hours either side HW
Restrictions:	8 knot speed limit within 400m shore: this is a desig-nated water-skiing area, other activities are not permit-ted; to gain access you must join the T.D.C. Water Safety Group - contact number above for details
Facilities:	fuel nearby, parking for car and trailer on site

Dues:	none
Charge:	none
Directions:	from Canterbury follow A28 east: at Birchington town square take Station Rd to Minnis Bay then turn right along Coast Rd towards Margate; site is at end of Beach Avenue
Waters accessed:	Thames Estuary

Margate - Minnis Bay, Birchington
Tel: (01843) 577529 (Foreshore Manager)

Type:	wide concrete slipway onto firm sand: beware soft sand & mud at LW
Suits:	all craft except pwc and speed boats
Availability:	approx. 2 hours either side HW
Restrictions:	8 knot speed limit within 400m shore: pwc, water-skiing and speed boats prohibited; to gain access you need to belong to the T.D.C. Water Safety Group - contact number above
Facilities:	fuel nearby, parking for car and trailer (c), toilets, pub and cafe
Dues:	none
Charge:	none
Directions:	from Canterbury follow A28 east: at Birchington town square take Station Rd to Minnis Bay: site is on the Parade
Waters accessed:	Thames Estuary

Herne Bay - Neptune Jetty Ramp, Central Parade
Tel: (01227) 264444 (Foreshore Manager)

Type:	wide medium concrete ramp into harbour
Suits:	small powered craft and pwc
Availability:	approx. 3 hours either side HW
Restrictions:	8 knot speed limit within 300m of shore: water-skiing permitted outside this area; site is exposed in northerly winds
Facilities:	fuel nearby, limited parking for car and trailer (c) on site, toilets nearby,other facilities 3 miles: water safety patrol boat in operation
Dues:	none
Charge:	none
Directions:	leave M2 at junction 7 and follow A299 to Herne Bay then signs to seafront; site is east of Pier near Clock Tower
Waters accessed:	Thames Estuary

Herne Bay - Breakwater Slipway, Central Parade
Tel: (01227) 264444 (Foreshore Manager)

Type:	gentle wide concrete ramp
Suits:	all craft up to 25'/7.6m LOA
Availability:	approx. 3 hours either side HW

Restrictions:	8 knot speed limit in harbour and within 300m of shore: water-skiing permitted outside this area; pwc permitted at this site only if there is a northerly wind at Neptune Jetty ramp
Facilities:	fuel nearby, parking for car and trailer (c) on site, toilets nearby, other facilities 3 miles: water safety patrol boat in operation
Dues:	none
Charge:	none
Directions:	leave M2 at junction 7 and follow A299 to Herne Bay then signs to seafront: site is east of Pier near Clock Tower
Waters accessed:	Thames Estuary

Herne Bay - Hampton Slipway, Swalecliffe Avenue
Tel: (01227) 264444 (Foreshore Manager)

Type:	gentle concrete and wood slipway with stepped slope onto mud and shingle beach
Suits:	small powered craft, sailing craft, ski-boats and pwc
Availability:	approx. 2½ hours either side HW
Restrictions:	8 knot speed limit within 300m of shore: this is a designated water-ski area with buoyed access lane from slipway; to the west of this lane is a designated pwc lane; site is exposed in northerly winds
Facilities:	fuel from garage nearby, parking for car and trailer and toilets on site, other facilities 3 miles: water safety patrol boat in operation
Dues:	none
Charge:	none
Directions:	follow B2205 west from Herne Bay, turning after 1½ miles from Hampton Pier Ave into Swalecliffe Ave
Waters accessed:	Thames Estuary

Whitstable Harbour - West Quay Slipway
Tel: (01227) 274086 (Harbour Master)

Type:	gentle timber ramp onto shingle/mud foreshore
Suits:	all craft
Availability:	approx. 3 hours either side HW
Restrictions:	8 knot speed limit within 300m of shore; site is exposed in N winds
Facilities:	fuel from garage (¼ mile), very limited parking by ramp (c) but large free car park opp. harbour (200m), toilets nearby, chandlery and outboard repairs (100m): water safety patrol boat in operation
Dues:	none
Charge:	none
Direction:	leave M2 at junction 7 following A299 to Whitstable then turn off towards sea and follow coast road to Harbour
Waters accessed:	Thames Estuary

Whitstable - Sea Wall (The Dinghy Store)

Tel: (01227) 274168

Type:	concrete slipway onto shingle
Suits:	all craft including pwc and windsurfers
Availability:	approx. 3 hours either side HW
Restrictions:	8 knot speed limit within 300m of shore: water-skiing permitted outside this area
Facilities:	fuel nearby, parking for car and trailer and toilets nearby, chandlery and outboard repairs available on site
Dues:	none
Charge:	none
Directions:	from M2 follow A299/A290: site is on sea wall just west of harbour
Waters accessed:	Thames Estuary

Conyer (The Swale) - Swale Marina, Conyer Wharf, Teynham

Tel: (0468) 347055

Type:	shallow concrete slipway
Suits:	all craft except pwc
Availability:	approx. 2 hours either side HW by prior arrangement
Restrictions:	8 knot speed limit inshore: water-skiing & pwc prohibited
Facilities:	diesel on site, parking for car and trailer, toilets and showers, chandlery and other boatyard facilities all on site
Dues:	none
Charge:	approx. £5
Directions:	from Sittingbourne follow A2 east, turning off onto minor roads and following signs to Teynham and then Conyer
Waters accessed:	Conyer Creek, The Swale and Thames Estuary

Sittingbourne (The Swale) - Kingsferry Bridge

Tel: (01795) 511116 (Long Reach Ski Club)

Type:	concrete ramp
Suits:	powered craft: members only
Availability:	at all states of tide
Restrictions:	launching is for members only
Facilities:	toilets & showers, parking for car and trailer on site: other facilities in Sittingbourne (4 miles)
Dues:	none
Charge:	yes - on application
Directions:	leave M2 at junction 5 following A249 to Sheerness and follow signs to Ridham Dock: site is on mainland side of bridge
Waters accessed:	The Swale and Thames Estuary

Queenborough, Isle of Sheppey - Queenborough Hard, High Street
Tel: (01795) 662051 (Swale Borough Council)

Type:	shallow narrow concrete slipway (approx. 7'/2m wide) over mud
Suits:	all craft up to 20'/6.1m LOA except pwc
Availability:	all states of tide
Restrictions:	8 knot speed limit in harbour: water-skiing permitted in Long Reach designated area only; diving permitted outside harbour area; pwc prohibited; access road to site is narrow
Facilities:	fuel nearby, parking for car and trailer nearby, chandlery and toilets on site, outboard repairs, shops, pubs and restaurants nearby: moorings and temporary membership Queenborough Y.C. available
Dues:	none
Charge:	approx. £5
Directions:	leave M2 at junction 5 following A249 to Sheerness: after Kingsferry Br follow signs to Queenborough and signs to harbour
Waters accessed:	The Swale, River Medway and Thames Estuary

Sheerness, Isle of Sheppey - Barton Point, Marine Parade

Type:	steep concrete ramp
Suits:	small sailing and powered craft only: no pwc
Availability:	approx. 2 hours either side HW
Restrictions:	8 knot speed limit inshore: water-skiing permitted in designated area offshore with access lane
Facilities:	parking for car and trailer, toilets and Sheppey Y.C. adjacent
Dues:	none
Charge:	none
Direction:	leave M2 at junction 5 following A249 to Isle of Sheppey and signs to Sheerness: access to site is via Marine Parade
Waters accessed:	Thames Estuary

Minstor, Isle of Sheppey - Minstor Shingle Bank Slipway
Tel: (01795) 667015 (Swale Borough Council)

Type:	shallow concrete ramp approx. 10'/3m wide onto shingle
Suits:	small craft only: no pwc
Availability:	approx. 2 hours either side HW
Restrictions:	8 knot speed limit inshore: water-skiing permitted in designated area; pwc prohibited; site exposed in onshore winds
Facilities:	parking for car and trailer (c), toilets nearby; Minstor Windsurf Club is based here
Dues:	none
Charge:	none
Directions:	leave M2 at junction 5 and follow A249 to Sheerness: at Clock Tower turn right onto Marine Parade and follow for 1 1/4 miles
Waters accessed:	Thames Estuary

Gillingham (River Medway) - Commodore Hard, The Strand

Type:	long narrow concrete slipway
Suits:	sailing dinghies and other small craft which can be manhandled
Availability:	all states of tide
Restrictions:	6 knot speed limit in river: water-skiing and pwc are prohibited; access via narrow road and vehicles are not permitted on slipway
Facilities:	fuel nearby, limited parking for car only in public car parks 250-300m away (these car parks can become very congested); no parking for trailers, toilets on site, chandlery nearby
Dues:	none
Charge:	none
Directions:	leave M2 at junction 4 following A278 to A2 and turn right; turn left onto B2004 (Lower Rainham Road) and site is accessed from this road
Waters accessed:	River Medway, The Swale and Thames Estuary

Gillingham (River Medway) - Gillingham Marina, Pier Road
Tel: (01634) 280022

Type:	two boat hoists (up to 65 tons) into locked marina basin
Suits:	larger craft only
Availability:	weekday daylight hours by arrangement only: contact the Berthing Manager; access to river via lock approx. 4 hours either side HW
Restrictions:	6 knot speed limit in river
Facilities:	fuel, parking for car and trailer, toilets and showers, chandlery and other marina facilities on site
Dues:	none
Charge:	approx. £9 + vat per metre for launch and recovery
Directions:	leave M2 at junction 4 following A278 to A2 and turning right; turn left onto B2004, site is accessed via Pier Rd
Waters accessed:	River Medway, The Swale and Thames Estuary

Halling (River Medway) - Elmhaven Marina, Rochester Rd
Tel: (01634) 240489

Type:	steep concrete slipway
Suits:	all craft
Availability:	approx. 2 hours either side HW during normal working hours by prior arrangement
Restrictions:	6 knot speed limit in river: water-skiing and pwc prohibited: site is above Rochester Bridge where there is restricted headroom and access is via a narrow gate (9' 10"/ 3m wide)
Facilities:	parking for car and trailer (c), toilets, showers and marine engineer on site
Dues:	none
Charge:	approx. £8 per metre

| Directions: | leave M2 at junction 2 following A228 south through Cuxton |
| Waters accessed: | River Medway, The Swale and Thames Estuary |

Cuxton (River Medway) - Cuxton Marina, Station Road

Tel: (01634) 721941

Type:	concrete slipway
Suits:	dinghies and small powered craft
Availability:	approx. 2 hours either side HW during normal working hours by prior arrangement
Restrictions:	6 knot speed limit: water-skiing and pwc prohibited; site is above Rochester Bridge and there is restricted headroom
Facilities:	parking for car and trailer, toilets and outboard repairs on site, chandlery nearby
Dues:	none
Charge:	approx. £5
Directions:	leave M2 at junction 2 and follow A228 south through Cuxton: marina is on left
Waters accessed:	River Medway

Rochester (River Medway) - Medway Bridge Marina, Manor Lane

Tel: (01634) 843576

Type:	launching by marina equipment only
Suits:	all craft up to 16 tons
Availability:	0900-1700 weekdays only by prior arrangement
Restrictions:	6 knot speed limit in river
Facilities:	fuel, parking for car and trailer, toilets, showers, chandlery, repairs, restaurant, bar all on site
Dues:	none
Charge:	approx. £31 + vat
Directions:	leave M2 at junction 23 and follow signs to Borstal in Rochester direction. Turn left into Priestfields and after nearly 1 mile turn right down Manor Lane; marina is at bottom of steep hill
Waters accessed:	River Medway, The Swale and Thames Estuary

Gravesend (River Thames) - Gravesham Marina, Gravesend Promenade

Tel: (01474) 352392

Type:	shallow concrete ramp with winch & crane up to 9 tonnes
Suits:	all craft except pwc and windsurfers
Availability:	at all states of tide: lock into river opens from 1 hour before to HW
Restrictions:	3 knot speed limit in marina: locked barrier, key from lockkeeper
Facilities:	diesel on site, petrol nearby, parking for car and trailer, toilets, outboard repairs and secure compound on site; chandlery and diving supplies nearby
Dues:	approx. £6.50

Charge:	tide fee (approx. £6) charged for lock opening before 0700 and after 2100 due to tide times
Directions:	from London take A2 following signs to Rochester: at Gravesend east turn off along Valley Drive, turning right into Old Rd East: at roundabout turn left along Rochester Rd to next roundabout then right into Ordnance Rd: site is at bottom of road
Waters accessed:	River Thames

Basildon (River Thames) - Wat Tyler Country Park Marina, Pitsea Hall Lane
Tel: (01268) 550088/583681

Type:	steep concrete slipway
Suits:	craft up to 30'/9m LOA
Availability:	approx. 2½ hours either side HW from 0800 to dusk
Restrictions:	8 knot speed limit: water-skiing and pwc permitted in designated areas; no windsurfing; 3rd party insurance certificate required; locked gate opened on payment of launch fee
Facilities:	fuel (1 mile), parking for car and trailer, toilets, cafe, chandlery, storage ashore, visitor's moorings & motor boat museum on site
Dues:	none
Charge:	approx. £10.20
Directions:	follow A 13 from London to Basildon, turning off to follow signs to Country Park
Waters accessed:	Vange Ck,Holehaven Ck and Thames Estuary

South Benfleet (River Thames) - Benfleet Causeway

Type:	two concrete slipways, one either side of Benfleet Ck barrage
Suits:	all craft
Availability:	approx. 2 hours either side HW
Restrictions:	8 knot speed limit: water-skiing permitted in designated areas at some distance from this site: pwc prohibited
Facilities:	parking for car and trailer nearby (c), toilets, chandlery and outboard repairs nearby
Dues:	none
Charge:	none
Directions:	from Southend follow A127/A13 west towards London: take A130 south to Canvey Island: on island take first left back to Benfleet: sites are immediately on right hand side over bridge
Waters accessed:	Benfleet Creek and Thames Estuary

Leigh-on-Sea - Two Tree Island
Tel: (01702) 711010

Type:	concrete slipway
Suits:	all craft
Availability:	approx. 4 hours either side HW
Restrictions:	8 knot speed limit: pwc prohibited; water-skiing permitted

	in designated areas nearby
Facilities:	parking for car and trailer and toilets on site, chandlery and outboard repairs nearby
Dues:	none
Charge:	approx. £9.95
Directions:	from Southend follow A13 to Leigh-on-Sea, turning off at railway station into Marsh Rd: site is approx. 1 mile down road
Waters accessed:	Thames Estuary

Leigh-on-Sea - Old High Street

Tel: (01702) 710561

Type:	concrete slipway
Suits:	dinghies and small trailer-sailers
Availability:	approx. 2 hours either side HW
Restrictions:	8 knot speed limit: water-skiing permitted in designated areas; pwc prohibited; access is via narrow busy High St
Facilities:	fuel nearby, parking for car nearby (c), no parking for trailer, toilets on site, chandlery and outboard repairs nearby in 'Old Leigh'
Dues:	none
Charge:	none
Directions:	from Southend follow A13 four miles to Leigh Old Town turning off 400m from railway station
Waters accessed:	Thames Estuary

Southend-on-Sea - Esplanade

Tel: (01702) 611889 (Foreshore Office, Pier Hill)

Type:	concrete slipway onto sand
Suits:	small craft which can be manhandled
Availability:	approx. 2½ hours either side HW
Restrictions:	8 knot speed limit: water-skiing permitted in designated areas; pwc prohibited; access is via busy seafront road
Facilities:	fuel nearby, parking for car and trailer in local car parks (c), chandlery, diving supplies and outboard repairs nearby
Dues:	none
Charge:	none
Directions:	from London follow A13 or A127 to Southend then signs to seafront: site is 1 mile east of Pier
Waters accessed:	Thames Estuary

Shoeburyness - West Beach

Tel: (01702) 293742

Type:	steep concrete slipway onto hard sand
Suits:	all craft except pwc
Availability:	approx. 3 hours either side HW

Restrictions:	8 knot speed limit: water-skiing permitted in buoyed area with access corridor; pwc are prohibited
Facilities:	parking for car (c) in public car park nearby and for trailer (c) on site, toilets nearby
Dues:	none
Charge:	approx. £9.95
Directions:	follow A13 four miles east of Southend: site is on seafront opposite the end of Waterford Rd and adjacent Coastguard Station
Waters accessed:	Thames Estuary

Shoeburyness - East Beach Road

Tel: (01702) 293744

Type:	concrete slipway onto hard sand
Suits:	all craft
Availability:	approx. 4 hours either side HW 0900-1600
Restrictions:	8 knot speed limit: water-skiing permitted in buoyed area with access corridor
Facilities:	parking for car and trailer (c) on site, toilets
Dues:	none
Charge:	approx. £9.95
Directions:	from Southend follow A13 east for about 5 miles: site is on seafront with access through East Beach car park
Waters accessed:	Thames Estuary

Paglesham (River Roach) - Paglesham Boatyard Ltd, East End

Tel: (01702) 258885

Type:	shallow concrete ramp to centre of river
Suits:	all craft
Availability:	all states of tide during daylight hours
Restrictions:	8 knot speed limit through moorings: water-skiing permitted in designated areas in River Crouch; sea wall gate closed at night
Facilities:	petrol nearby, diesel, parking for car and trailer, toilets, crane, cafe, overnight moorings all on site, chandlery & pub nearby
Dues:	none
Charge:	approx. £5 (put through letterbox if nobody in yard)
Directions:	from Southend follow A127 west turning onto B1013 to Rochford: turn onto minor roads following signs to Stambridge, then East End, Paglesham; follow unmade road from Plough and Sail pub
Waters accessed:	River Roach, River Crouch and Thames Estuary

Wallasea Island (River Crouch) - Essex Marina, Canewdon

Tel: (01702) 258531

Type:	shallow concrete ramp
Suits:	all craft
Availability:	during working hours (0800 - 1800) daily by prior arrangement
Restrictions:	8 knot speed limit near marina

Facilities:	fuel, parking for car and trailer, toilets & showers, chandlery, bar, restaurant and other marina facilities all on site
Dues:	approx. £11.50 p.a.(contact Harbour Office Tel: 01621 783602)
Charge:	approx. £16
Directions:	from London follow A12/A127 to Rayleigh then A129/B1013 north: at Hockley turn onto minor roads following signs to Canewdon
Waters accessed:	River Crouch and Thames Estuary

Hullbridge Ford (River Crouch) - Ferry Road

Tel: (01621) 783602 (Harbour Office, The Quay, Burnham-on-Crouch)

Type:	launching from tarmac road onto shingle
Suits:	dinghies and small powered craft
Availability:	approx. 2 hours either side HW
Restrictions:	8 knot speed limit: water-skiing permitted but only by special licence; access is via a narrow road and slipway is not maintained below mean HW level
Facilities:	parking for car and trailer (c) on site
Dues:	approx. £11.50 p.a.
Charge:	no additional fee
Directions:	from Chelmsford follow A130 south, turning off through Battlesbridge onto minor roads and following signs: site is on south bank of river
Waters accessed:	River Crouch and Thames Estuary

South Woodham Ferrers (River Crouch)

Tel: (01621) 783602 (Harbour Office, The Quay, Burnham-on-Crouch)

Type:	launching over poor shingle and mud surface
Suits:	dinghies and small powered craft
Availability:	approx. 2 hours either side HW
Restrictions:	8 knot speed limit: water-skiing permitted but only by special licence; access is via a narrow road and slipway is not maintained
Facilities:	parking for car and trailer (c) on site
Dues:	approx. £11.50 p.a.
Charge:	none
Directions:	from Chelmsford follow A130 south, turning east onto A132/B1012 and following road past station: site is on north bank of river in Country Park opposite Hullbridge
Waters accessed:	River Crouch and Thames Estuary

Burnham-on-Crouch (River Crouch) - Burnham Yacht Harbour

Tel: (01621) 782150

Type:	concrete slipway, 30 ton travel hoist and crane
Suits:	all craft except speedboats
Availability:	all states of tide during daylight hours
Restrictions:	8 knot speed limit: water-skiing, speedboats and pwc prohibited

Facilities:	diesel, parking for car and trailer, toilets and showers, chandlery and other marina facilities on site
Dues:	approx. £11.50 p.a.(contact Harbour Office Tel: (01621) 783602)
Charge:	approx. £6
Directions:	from Chelmsford follow A130 south, turning onto A132/B1012 and following B1010 east to Burnham-on-Crouch: cross over railway bridge and turn right by shops into Foundry Lane
Waters accessed:	River Crouch and Thames Estuary

Bradwell-on-Sea (River Blackwater) - Bradwell Marina, Waterside

Tel: (01621) 776391

Type:	two medium concrete ramps
Suits:	all craft except pwc & windsurfers
Availability:	approx. 4½ hours either side HW after 0830
Restrictions:	8 knot speed limit: all boats must be able to leave and return to marina under power, pwc are prohibited: water-skiing is permitted in river in designated areas; locked barrier to site
Facilities:	fuel, parking for car and trailer, toilets and showers, chandlery, other marina facilities and clubhouse available to visitors on site
Dues:	none
Charge:	approx. £10-£12 depending on type of craft
Directions:	from Chelmsford follow A414 to Maldon, then B1018 south to Latchingdon: turn left onto signposted minor roads
Waters accessed:	River Blackwater and Thames Estuary

Maylandsea (River Blackwater) - Blackwater Marina, Marine Parade

Tel: (01621) 740264

Type:	wide shallow concrete slipway
Suits:	all craft
Availability:	approx. 2-3 hours either side HW 0900-1600 by prior arrangement with marina office
Restrictions:	8 knot speeed limit in river: water-skiing,windsurfing and pwc permitted in designated areas
Facilities:	diesel on site, petrol nearby, parking for car and trailer, toilets and showers, full workshop and bar/club/restaurant all on site
Dues:	none
Charge:	approx. £10
Directions:	from Chelmsford follow A414 to Maldon, then B1018 south to Latchingdon: turn left onto signposted minor roads and left again after approx. 2½ miles
Waters accessed:	River Blackwater and Thames Estuary

Little Baddow (Chelmer & Blackwater Navigation) - Paper Mill Lock
Tel: (01245) 223482 (Chelmer & Blackwater Nav. Ltd.)

Type:	shallow concrete ramp
Suits:	all powered craft
Availability:	by prior arrangement only
Restrictions:	4 mph speed limit on canal: site gives access to locked waterway and open sea at Maldon (14 miles)
Facilities:	parking for car and trailer on site, toilets, and outboard repairs all on site
Dues:	none
Charge:	approx. £24
Directions:	from A12 take A414 to Maldon, turning left at Danbury Green to Little Baddow; go down the hill for 2½ miles and Lock House is just before river bridge
Waters accessed:	Chelmer & Blackwater Navigation and River Blackwater

Maldon (River Blackwater) - Promenade Park
Tel: (01621) 856487 (River Bailiff, Maldon D.C.)

Type:	concrete slipway onto soft mud
Suits:	small craft except pwc
Availability:	approx. 1 hour either side HW during daylight hours
Restrictions:	8 knot speed limit: no pwc; gate to park locked at night
Facilities:	fuel in town, parking for car and trailer (c) and toilets on site, chandlery nearby
Dues:	none
Charge:	none
Directions:	from Chelmsford take A414 to Maldon, following Maldon southern by-pass and signs to Promenade: site is at seaward end of park
Waters accessed:	River Blackwater and Thames Estuary

Maldon (River Blackwater) - Maldon Boatyard, North Street
Tel: (01206) 382244 (West Mersea Marine)

Type:	concrete slipway
Suits:	all craft except pwc
Availability:	approx. 2 hours either side HW
Restrictions:	8 knot speed limit: water-skiing permitted in designated areas downstream; pwc prohibited; site is locked at night
Facilities:	fuel nearby, parking for car and trailer on site, toilets, chandlery and shipwright on site
Dues:	none
Charge:	approx. £8
Directions:	from Chelmsford take A414 to Maldon High St: continue down High St turning left into North St; site is at bottom of street
Waters accessed:	River Blackwater and Thames Estuary

Tollesbury - Woodrolfe Boatyard, Tollesbury Marina

Tel: (01621) 869202

Type:	3 concrete slipways, steep and shallow
Suits:	all craft except pwc
Availability:	approx. 2 hours either side HW during daylight hours
Restrictions:	4 knot speed limit in Woodrolfe Ck, 8 knots in Tollesbury Fleet: check for availability before use; locked barrier at night
Facilities:	diesel on site, petrol nearby, parking for car and trailer, toilets and showers, crane, hoist, moorings and other marina facilities on site
Dues:	none
Charge:	approx. £7 + vat
Directions:	from Maldon take B1026 to Tolleshunt D'Arcy turning right onto B1023 to Tollesbury: after village fork left into Woodrolfe Rd
Waters accessed:	Woodrolfe Creek, Tollesbury Fleet and River Blackwater

Tollesbury - Tollesbury Saltings Ltd. The Sail Lofts, Woodrolfe Road

Tel: (01621) 868624

Type:	concrete ramp
Suits:	small sailing and powered craft
Availability:	approx. 2 hours either side HW 0830-1730 by prior arrangement
Restrictions:	8 knot speed limit: water-skiing and pwc permitted in designated areas in River Blackwater
Facilities:	fuel nearby, parking for car and trailer (c), toilets, chandlery, outboard repairs, yacht repairs & rigging all on site
Dues:	none
Charge:	approx. £5
Directions:	turn off A12 through Kelvedon onto B1024 (B1023) to Tiptree and then through Tolleshunt D'Arcy: in Tollesbury fork into Woodrolfe Rd; site is behind sail lofts by sea wall
Waters accessed:	Woodrolfe Creek, Tollesbury Fleet and River Blackwater

West Mersea - Public Hard, Coast Road (previously 'Lifeboat Hard')

Tel: (01206) 382244

Type:	wide concrete and shingle hard
Suits:	all craft
Availability:	approx. 3 hours either side HW
Restrictions:	speed limit through moorings: water-skiing permitted in Strood Channel above moorings
Facilities:	fuel, limited parking for car and trailer, toilets and chandlery nearby
Dues:	none
Charge:	none

Directions:	from Colchester follow B1025 to Mersea Island and signs to West Mersea: follow road through village to waterfront
Waters accessed:	Blackwater Estuary

Rowhedge (River Colne) - Public Hard

Type:	concrete slipway onto mud
Suits:	small dinghies only
Availability:	approx. 1½ hours either side HW
Restrictions:	6 knot speed limit: water-skiing and pwc prohibited; awkward right-angled approach to slipway; site owned by Rowhedge Hard Assn.
Facilities:	fuel in village, limited parking for car and trailer in road, pub
Dues:	none
Charge:	none
Directions:	from Colchester follow Southway east, straight across roundabout by Colchester Town railway station then right fork into Military Road at traffic lights (signposted Rowhedge): continue following this road until left fork to Rowhedge: site is adjacent Anchor Inn
Waters accessed:	River Colne and Blackwater Estuary

Alresford (River Colne) - The Ford

Type:	shingle hard
Suits:	small craft
Availability:	approx. 2½ hours either side HW
Restrictions:	8 knot speed limit; water-skiing and pwc prohibited
Facilities:	limited parking for car and trailer
Dues:	none
Charge:	none
Directions:	from Colchester take A133 towards Clacton, turning right onto B1027 and at Alresford turn right into village: follow road past railway station and take road marked 'Ford'
Waters accessed:	Alresford Creek, River Colne and Blackwater Estuary

Brightlingsea (River Colne) - Town Hard
Tel: (01206) 302200 (Harbour Office)

Type:	concrete and shingle hard
Suits:	all craft
Availability:	all states of tide
Restrictions:	4 knot speed limit in creek: water-skiing in designated area for members of Brightlingsea Powerboat and Water Ski Club only
Facilities:	fuel, parking for car and trailer in Tower St or Oyster Tank Rd (c), toilets, chandlers and pub all available on site or nearby
Dues:	none
Charge:	yes

Directions:	from Colchester take A133 towards Clacton: turn right onto B1027 to Thorrington cross roads and turn right onto B1029; at Brightlingsea follow signs to 'Waterfront'
Waters accessed:	Brightlingsea Creek, River Colne and Blackwater Estuary

St Osyth (River Colne) - St Osyth Boatyard

Tel: (01255) 820005

Type:	concrete slipway
Suits:	dinghies and trailer-sailers
Availability:	approx. 2 hours either side HW during working hours by prior arrangement
Restrictions:	5 knot speed limit in creek: powered craft and pwc prohibited; creek is narrow and use is very limited by tide
Facilities:	parking for car and trailer nearby, toilets on site
Dues:	none
Charge:	approx. £3
Directions:	from Colchester take A133 towards Clacton, turning right onto B1027 near Essex University: turn right into St Osyth village turning right again past 'Priory' to creek: site is on right
Waters accessed:	St Osyth Creek, River Colne and Blackwater Estuary

Clacton-on-Sea - Martello Bay, Hastings Avenue

Tel: (01255) 425501 (Tendring D.C.)

Type:	concrete ramp onto soft sand
Suits:	small craft which can be manhandled
Availability:	at all states of tide over beach
Restrictions:	8 knot speed limit within 200m of LW mark: launch into buoyed channel; water-skiing, pwc & windsurfing permitted outside this area; no vehicles permitted on beach
Facilities:	fuel in town, parking for car & trailer(c), toilets nearby, chandlery & outboard repairs in Walton
Dues:	none
Charge:	none
Directions:	from Colchester follow A133 to Clacton then signs to seafront: site is 1 mile west of Pier
Waters accessed:	Thames Estuary and North Sea

Clacton-on-Sea - Holland Haven, Holland-on-Sea

Tel: (01255) 425501 (Tendring D.C.)

Type:	concrete slipway onto sand
Suits:	dinghies only
Availability:	approx. 3 hours either side HW
Restrictions:	8 knot speed limit within 200m of LW mark: water-skiing permitted outside this area
Facilities:	parking for car and trailer (c), toilets, Clacton-on-Sea S.C. adjacent

Dues:	none
Charge:	none
Directions:	from Colchester follow A133 to Clacton then B1032 to Holland-on-Sea and signs to seafront: access is from Esplanade
Waters accessed:	Thames Estuary and North Sea

Frinton-on-Sea - The Esplanade

Tel: (01255) 425501 (Tendring D.C.)

Type:	concrete slipway onto hard sand
Suits:	all craft
Availability:	approx. 3 hours either side HW
Restrictions:	8 knot speed limit inshore: water-skiing permitted outside limit; access is via locked barrier, key from Beach Attendant or Council Offices, Old Rd, Frinton
Facilities:	fuel in town, parking for car and trailer (c) on site and toilets nearby, chandlers in town
Dues:	none
Charge:	none
Directions:	from Colchester follow A133 and B1033 turning right at station over level crossing and follow signs to seafront
Waters accessed:	Thames Estuary and North Sea

Walton-on-the-Naze - Town Hard, Mill Lane

Type:	launching over shingle foreshore
Suits:	all craft up to 20'/6.1m LOA
Availability:	approx. 1½ hours either side HW
Restrictions:	8 knot speed limit: water-skiing prohibited
Facilities:	fuel, parking for car and trailer(c), toilets, boatyard and chandlers nearby
Dues:	none
Charge:	none
Directions:	from Colchester follow A133/B1033: turn left onto B1034 after Thorpe-le-Soken and left again off High St into Mill Lane
Waters accessed:	Walton Backwaters and Thames Estuary

Walton-on-the-Naze - Titchmarsh Marina, Coles Lane, Kirby Road

Tel: (01255) 851899

Type:	shallow concrete ramp
Suits:	sailing and small powered craft up to 25'/7.6m LOA
Availability:	all states of tide 0830-2000 during season
Restrictions:	8 knot speed limit: no speed boats, pwc or wind-surfers; locked security gates out of hours
Facilities:	diesel on site, petrol nearby, parking for car and trailer, toilets, chandlery, outboard repairs, crane, travel lift, rigging service, restaurant and bar all on site
Dues:	none
Charge:	approx. £10

Directions:	from Colchester follow A133/B1033: turn left onto B1034 after Thorpe-le-Soken and left at sign at approach to town
Waters accessed:	Walton Backwaters and Thames Estuary

Dovercourt - Seafront

Type:	concrete slipway onto sand
Suits:	all craft
Availability:	approx. 2 hours either side HW
Restrictions:	8 knot speed limit in harbour, water-skiing permitted in designated area clear of shipping channel
Facilities:	fuel in town, parking for car and trailer (c), toilets
Dues:	none
Charge:	none
Directions:	from Colchester take A1232 towards Ipswich and then A120 east to Harwich: follow signs to Dovercourt and seafront and site is adjacent boating lake
Waters accessed:	Harwich Harbour and Thames Estuary

Harwich - Kings Quay Slip, Wellington Road

Type:	concrete slipway onto shingle
Suits:	all craft
Availability:	all states of tide for small boats: approx. 3 hours either side HW for larger craft
Restrictions:	8 knot speed limit: no water-skiing in harbour; this is a busy commercial harbour and craft must keep clear of deep-water channel and ferry terminals
Facilities:	fuel nearby, parking for car and trailer, toilets, chandlery all nearby
Dues:	none
Charge:	none
Directions:	from Colchester take A1232 towards Ipswich and then A120 east to Harwich: site is accessed via Kings Quay St and is adjacent to Harwich Town S.C.
Waters accessed:	Harwich Harbour and Thames Estuary

Manningtree (River Stour) - Quay St

Type:	fairly steep concrete slipway
Suits:	small craft
Availability:	approx. 2 hours either side HW
Restrictions:	speed limit: water-skiing permitted in designated area downstream
Facilities:	fuel nearby, parking for car and trailer in road, toilets nearby
Dues:	none
Charge:	none
Directions:	from Colchester follow A137, turning right at round-about near Manningtree Railway Station and left at end of High St: site is opposite Stour S.C.
Waters accessed:	River Stour, Harwich Harbour and North Sea

Brantham (River Stour) - Cattawade Street

Type:	concrete slipway with rollers and hand winch
Suits:	small craft that can be manhandled
Availability:	approx 1½ hours either side HW for launching into tidal river or at all times for launching into non-tidal waterway
Restrictions:	speed limit: non-tidal river only suitable for small boats without masts; winch on slipway is locked, key from Sluice Keeper - see notice; no direct vehicular access to slipway
Facilities:	fuel nearby, limited parking for car and trailer, no toilets, pub and restaurant nearby
Dues:	none
Charge:	none
Directions:	from Colchester follow A137 north: after crossing river turn right and right again into Cattawade St; site is to left of old bridge past cottages
Waters accessed:	tidal and non-tidal River Stour and Harwich Harbour

Pin Mill (River Orwell) - Foreshore

Type:	launching over gently sloping shingle foreshore
Suits:	small craft only
Availability:	approx. 2-3 hours either side HW
Restrictions:	6 knot speed limit: water-skiing in designated area east of Levington Marina; beware commercial traffic in main channel; access road is narrow
Facilities:	fuel, parking for car and trailer (c), toilets, chandlery, boatyard facilities nearby, pub
Dues:	none
Charge:	none
Directions:	from Ipswich take A137, turning left at roundabout onto B1456: follow road to Chelmondiston and turn left to Pin Mill; site is opposite end of road
Waters accessed:	River Orwell and Harwich Harbour

Woolverstone (River Orwell) - Woolverstone Marina

Tel: (01473) 780206

Type:	steep concrete ramp
Suits:	small craft except pwc & windsurfers: trailer-sailers by prior arrangement only
Availability:	approx. 3-4 hours either side HW
Restrictions:	6 knot speed limit in river: water-skiing in designated area downstream but pwc prohibited: contact marina office prior to launching
Facilities:	diesel on site, parking for car and trailer, toilets and showers, chandlery and outboard repairs, launderette, club and restaurant
Dues:	none
Charge:	approx. £19
Directions:	from Ipswich (A137) take B1456 towards Shotley: in Woolverstone village turn left down long concrete drive at sign to marina
Waters accessed:	River Orwell and Harwich Harbour

Levington (River Orwell) - Suffolk Yacht Harbour

Tel: (01473) 659240

Type:	steep concrete ramp
Suits:	all craft except pwc
Availability:	all states of tide by prior arrangement
Restrictions:	6 knot speed limit in river: pwc prohibited; water-skiing permitted in designated area
Facilities:	fuel, parking for car and trailer, toilets, chandlery and outboard repairs, restaurant & club all available on site
Dues:	none
Charge:	approx. £8
Directions:	from Ipwich take A14 to Felixstowe turning right at sign to marina: site is on north bank of river
Waters accessed:	River Orwell and Harwich Harbour

Felixstowe - The Dip, Cliff Road

Tel: (01394) 444323 (Suffolk Coastal D.C.)

Type:	concrete slipway onto shingle beach
Suits:	sailing craft only
Availability:	approx. 2 hours either side HW
Restrictions:	no powered craft; gate in sea wall may be closed in winter
Facilities:	fuel in town, parking for car (c) on site but not for trailer, toilets
Dues:	none
Charge:	none
Directions:	from Ipswich follow A14 going straight on at roundabout at approach to town and again at next roundabout: turn right at 3rd roundabout into Beatrice Avenue and left into High Rd East at next roundabout; site is on right after Brackenbury Fort car park
Waters accessed:	North Sea

Felixstowe Ferry (River Deben)

Type:	steep cobblestone ramp onto shingle foreshore
Suits:	small craft
Availability:	all states of tide but approx. 4 hours either side HW for larger boats; priority at all times to be given to boatyard
Restrictions:	8 knot speed limit: water-skiing in designated area under control of East Suffolk Water Ski Club; larger craft should contact Felixstowe Ferry Boatyard Tel: (01394) 282173
Facilities:	diesel on site, petrol nearby, limited turning, no parking for car and trailer, toilets and chandlery on site, outboard repairs nearby; cafe, sailing club with showers, bar etc
Dues:	none
Charge:	approx. £8 for craft under 30hp, £12 for craft over 30hp

Directions:	from Ipswich follow A14 going straight on at round-about at approach to town and again at next round-about: turn right at 3rd roundabout into Beatrice Avenue and left into High Rd East: follow road across golf course to ferry
Waters accessed:	River Deben and North Sea

Waldringfield (River Deben) - Foreshore

Type:	short narrow concrete slipway with drop onto shingle and broken concrete
Suits:	sailing dinghies
Availability:	approx. 2 hours either side HW
Restrictions:	8 knot speed limit in river: narrow access road and limited room to manoeuvre trailers etc.
Facilities:	fuel in village, parking for car and trailer nearby through pub car park, toilets nearby, chandlery adjacent
Dues:	none
Charge:	none
Directions:	from Woodbridge follow A12: turn left at roundabout after Martlesham Heath to Waldringfield and site is on west bank of river, in front of Maybush Inn
Waters accessed:	River Deben

Woodbridge (River Deben) - Robertsons Boatyard, Lime Kiln Quay

Tel: (01394) 382305

Type:	shallow concrete ramp
Suits:	all craft except pwc and ski-boats
Availability:	approx. 2 hours either side HW by prior arrangement during working hours
Restrictions:	8 knot speed limit in river: water-skiing and pwc pro-hibited; check for availability
Facilities:	diesel on site, petrol in town, limited parking for car and trailer on site but public car park nearby (c), chandlery nearby; access is via narrow road with tight bend
Dues:	none
Charge:	approx. £20
Directions:	from Ipswich take A12 and follow signs to Woodbridge: follow road, turning right at sharp left-hand bend before traffic lights; turn right over level crossing and then immediately right again and boat-yard is on left
Waters accessed:	River Deben

Orford (River Ore) - Town Quay

Type:	concrete slipway with drop at end
Suits:	all craft up to 20'/6.1m LOA except pwc
Availability:	all states of tide: launching licence is required
Restrictions:	5 knot speed limit through moorings: water-skiing per-mitted in designated area by licence; priority given to members of Alde & Ore Water Ski Club; pwc prohibited

Facilities:	diesel on site, parking for car and trailer nearby (c), toilets nearby, chandlery and outboard repairs on site, moorings
Dues:	none
Charge:	approx. £3 per day (£35 p.a.); powered craft over 15hp - £20 per day (£80 p.a.)
Directions:	from Ipswich follow A12, turning onto A1152 at round-about north of Woodbridge and forking right onto B1084 following signs to Orford: site is at end of village street
Waters accessed:	River Ore and River Alde

Aldeburgh (River Alde) - Slaughden Quay (R. F. Upson & Co)
Tel: (01728) 453047

Type:	concrete slipway onto shingle
Suits:	all craft
Availability:	all states of tide during working hours with permission
Restrictions:	speed limit; water-skiing permitted in designated areas
Facilities:	diesel on site, petrol nearby, parking for car and trailer nearby, toilets, chandlery and boatyard services on site
Dues:	approx. £3.50; speedboats approx. £10
Charge:	no separate fee charged
Directions:	from Ipswich follow A12 north; turn right onto A1094 to Aldeburgh
Waters accessed:	River Alde and River Ore

Southwold - Public Hard, Blackshore
Tel: (01502) 724712 (Harbour Master)

Type:	concrete slipway
Suits:	all craft
Availability:	approx. 4 hours either side HW
Restrictions:	4 knot speed limit in harbour: water-skiing permitted above bridge by licence only (contact Hb Mr)
Facilities:	diesel nearby, limited parking for car and trailer (contact Hb Mr), toilets, chandlery, pub and tearooms nearby
Dues:	approx. £4.50 daily; £31 p.a.
Charge:	no separate fee charged
Directions:	from Ipswich follow A12 north, turning onto A1095 after Blythburgh: turn right at 'Kings Head' and left at Quay: site is adjacent old lifeboat shed
Waters accessed:	River Blyth and North Sea

Southwold - Boatyard, Chandlery and Tearoom, Blackshore
Tel: (01502) 722593

Type:	medium concrete ramp
Suits:	all craft
Availability:	approx. 4 hours either side HW by prior arrangement
Restrictions:	4 knot speed limit in harbour: water-skiing permitted above bridge by licence only (contact Hb Mr)

Facilities:	diesel, limited parking for car and trailer, toilets nearby, chandlery, boat repairs and tearooms on site, pub nearby
Dues:	no separate fee charged
Charge:	approx. £3
Directions:	from Ipswich follow A12 north, turning onto A1095 after Blythburgh: turn right at 'Kings Head' and left at Quay; site is in front of chandlery/tearooms
Waters accessed:	River Blyth and North Sea

Hemsby - Beach

Type:	launching over sandy beach
Suits:	light craft which can be manhandled
Availability:	all states of tide
Restrictions:	8 knot speed limit inshore: water-skiing permitted outside limit; site suitable for use in settled conditions only; access and parking can be difficult at peak times
Facilities:	none
Dues:	none
Charge:	none
Directions:	from Gt Yarmouth follow A149 and B1159 north for about 6 miles: turn right to Hemsby and follow track to beach
Waters accessed:	North Sea

Winterton-on-Sea - Beach

Type:	launching over sandy foreshore
Suits:	light craft only
Availability:	all states of tide
Restrictions:	8 knot speed limit inshore; water-skiing permitted outside limit; site suitable for use in settled conditions only; access and parking can be difficult at peak times
Facilities:	none
Dues:	none
Charge:	none
Directions:	from Gt Yarmouth follow A149 and B1159 north for about 8 miles: turn right to Winterton and follow signs to beach
Waters accessed:	North Sea

Whimpwell Green - Cart Gap, Eccles Beach

Type:	wooden ramp onto soft sand
Suits:	small craft only
Availability:	approx. 2 hours either side HW
Restrictions:	8 knot speed limit inshore: water-skiing permitted outside limit; conditions can be dangerous here
Facilities:	parking for car and trailer, toilets (summer only)
Dues:	none
Charge:	none
Directions:	from Gt Yarmouth follow A149 north, then turn right onto B1151 and left onto B1159: follow signs to beach
Waters accessed:	North Sea

Happisburgh - Beach

Type:	wooden ramp onto beach
Suits:	small craft only
Availability:	approx. 2 hours either side HW
Restrictions:	8 knot speed limit inshore: water-skiing permitted outside limit; conditions can be dangerous here
Facilities:	limited parking for car and trailer, toilets (summer only)
Dues:	none
Charge:	none
Directions:	from Gt Yarmouth follow A149 north, then turn right onto B1151 and left onto B1159; turn off close to Lighthouse
Waters accessed:	North Sea

Walcott Gap - Beach

Type:	concrete slipway onto sand
Suits:	light craft only
Availability:	approx. 2 hours either side HW
Restrictions:	8 knot speed limit inshore: water-skiing permitted outside limit; no parking on slipway or beach; open sea conditions
Facilities:	fuel, parking for car and trailer, toilets
Dues:	none
Charge:	none
Directions:	from Gt Yarmouth follow A149 north, then turn right onto B1150 in N. Walsham and left onto B1159: site is opposite Caravan Park
Waters accessed:	North Sea

Bacton - Beach

Type:	launching over sandy foreshore
Suits:	light craft only
Availability:	approx. 2 hours either side HW
Restrictions:	8 knot speed limit inshore: water-skiing permitted outside limit; site suitable for use in settled conditions only
Facilities:	parking for car and trailer (200m), no other facilities
Dues:	none
Charge:	none
Directions:	from Gt Yarmouth follow A149 north, then turn right onto B1150 to coast in N. Walsham and follow signs to beach
Waters accessed:	North Sea

Mundesley/Trimingham - Beach Road

Type:	launching over sandy beach with ramps from road
Suits:	light craft only
Availability:	all states of tide
Restrictions:	8 knot speed limit inshore: water-skiing permitted outside limit; site suitable for use in settled conditions only; access and parking can be difficult

Facilities:	none
Dues:	none
Charge:	none
Directions:	from Gt Yarmouth follow A149 north to N. Walsham, turning onto B1145 to Mundesley, then B1159 towards Trimingham; follow signs to Vale Rd approx. 1km west of Mundesley
Waters accessed:	North Sea

Cromer

Type:	ramp onto beach
Suits:	small craft which can be manhandled
Availability:	all states of tide
Restrictions:	8 knot speed limit inshore: water-skiing permitted outside limit; site suitable for use in settled conditions only; access and parking can be difficult at peak times
Facilities:	fuel from local garages, very limited parking
Dues:	none
Charge:	none
Directions:	from Norwich take A140 north: site is adjacent old lifeboat station
Waters accessed:	North Sea

Cromer - East Runton Gap

Type:	steep concrete slipway onto shingle
Suits:	all craft
Availability:	approx. 2 hours either side HW
Restrictions:	8 knot speed limit inshore; water-skiing permitted outside limit; site used by local fishing boats which may block access
Facilities:	parking for car and trailer, toilets
Dues:	none
Charge:	none
Directions:	from Cromer take A149 north west for approx. 3 miles, turning off towards beach: site is close to Gap Caravan Park
Waters accessed:	North Sea

Cromer - West Runton

Type:	ramp onto sandy beach
Suits:	light craft only
Availability:	all states of tide
Restrictions:	8 knot speed limit inshore: water-skiing permitted outside limit; site suitable for use in settled conditions only
Facilities:	fuel nearby, parking for car and trailer
Dues:	none
Charge:	none
Directions:	from Cromer take A149 north west turning right onto road to foreshore which ends at ramp
Waters accessed:	North Sea

Blakeney - Blakeney Harbour Quay

Type:	three concrete slipways
Suits:	all craft
Availability:	approx. 2 hours either side HW
Restrictions:	8 knot speed limit in harbour; water-skiing permitted at west end of harbour
Facilities:	fuel, parking for car and trailer (c), toilets, chandlery and boatyard facilities nearby
Dues:	none
Charge:	none
Directions:	from Cromer follow A149 north west to Blakeney and then signs to Quay
Waters accessed:	North Sea

Blakeney - Morston

Type:	launching over shingle foreshore
Suits:	small craft
Availability:	approx. 3 hours either side HW
Restrictions:	8 knot speed limit in harbour; water-skiing permitted at west end of harbour
Facilities:	parking for car and trailer, toilets, chandlery and boatyard facilities nearby in village
Dues:	none
Charge:	none
Directions:	from Cromer follow A149 north west and then yellow sign to Quay west of Blakeney
Waters accessed:	North Sea

Wells-next-the-Sea - East Quay
Tel: (01328) 711646 (Wells Harbour Commission)

Type:	concrete ramp with slipway trolley
Suits:	all craft except pwc
Availability:	approx. 2 hours either side HW by prior arrangement
Restrictions:	5 mph speed limit in inner harbour, 8 mph and 15 mph in channel: water-skiing permitted outside harbour with day membership of club; windsurfing permitted with permit (£10); pwc prohibited; powered vessels over 15'/4.6m LOA must carry 3rd party insurance
Facilities:	diesel on site, petrol nearby, parking for car and trailer (c), toilets, chandlery and outboard repairs nearby
Dues:	£2.50 up to 15'/4.6m LOA; £5 over 15'/4.6m LOA
Charge:	no additional fee
Directions:	from Cromer take A149 north west, turning off and following signs to harbour; access road is narrow
Waters accessed:	North Sea

Wells-next-the-Sea - Beach Road
Tel: (01328) 711646 (Wells Harbour Commission)

Type:	concrete ramp
Suits:	small craft except pwc
Availability:	approx. 2 hours either side HW by prior arrangement
Restrictions:	5 mph speed limit in inner harbour, 8 mph and 15 mph in channel; water-skiing permitted in designated area with day membership of club; windsurfing permitted with permit (£10); pwc prohibited; powered vessels over 15'/4.6m LOA must carry 3rd party insurance
Facilities:	diesel on site, petrol nearby, parking for car and trailer (c), toilets, chandlery and all other facilities nearby
Dues:	approx. £2.50 up to 15'/4.6m LOA; £5 over 15'/4.6m LOA
Charge:	none
Directions:	from Cromer take A149 north west, turning off and following signs to harbour: Beach Rd is opposite the caravan site
Waters accessed:	North Sea

Burnham Overy Staithe
Tel: (01328) 738348 (Burnham Overy Boathouse)

Type:	steep concrete slipway onto shingle
Suits:	dinghies: no powerboats or pwc
Availability:	approx. 2 hours either side HW
Restrictions:	8 knot speed limit: powerboats and pwc prohibited; site can be very congested at peak times
Facilities:	petrol (2 miles), limited parking for car nearby but not for trailer, chandlery and outboard repairs on site
Dues:	none
Charge:	approx. £10
Directions:	from Hunstanton follow A149 east for approx. 12 miles: site is opposite Burnham Overy Boathouse
Waters accessed:	The Wash and North Sea

Brancaster Harbour - The Beach

Type:	launching over shingle (several sites in harbour)
Suits:	small boats
Availability:	approx. 2-3 hours either side HW
Restrictions:	6 knot speed limit in harbour: water-skiing allowed out-side limits; Harbour Master's permission needed to launch powerboats and windsurfing is restricted
Facilities:	fuel, parking for car and trailer (c), toilets, chandlery nearby
Dues:	none
Charge:	yes
Directions:	from Hunstanton follow A149 east, turning off to follow signs
Waters accessed:	The Wash and North Sea

Hunstanton - North Beach
Tel: (01485) 535150 (Resort Manager)

Type:	concrete slipway onto hard sand
Suits	sailing dinghies and windsurfers only
Availability:	all states of tide but best approx. 2-3 hours either side HW
Restrictions:	7 knot speed limit within 200m of HW mark; powered craft prohibited
Facilities:	fuel, parking for car and trailer (c), toilets
Dues:	none
Charge:	none
Directions:	turn off A149: site is adjacent Pier and S.C.
Waters accessed:	The Wash and North Sea

Hunstanton - South Beach Road (Hunstanton Watersports Club)
Tel: (01485) 535827 (cafe) or (01485) 535940 (clubhouse)

Type:	concrete slipway onto hard sand
Suits	powered craft and pwc only
Availability:	approx. 3 hours either side HW 0900-1800
Restrictions:	8 mph speed limit inshore: certificate of 3rd party insurance required
Facilities:	fuel nearby, parking for car and trailer (c), toilets, out-board repairs, cafe, showers, licensed bar on site; changing rooms on site for club members only
Dues:	none
Charge:	approx. £10
Directions:	from Kings Lynn take A149 north to Hunstanton; at 1st roundabout turn left and head for coast, turning into South Beach Road
Waters accessed:	The Wash and North Sea

Hunstanton - Heacham Beach North
Tel: (01485) 535150 (Resort Manager)

Type:	launching over sand with tractor assistance
Suits	all craft up to 20'/6.1m LOA
Availability:	approx. 2-3 hours either side HW
Restrictions:	speed limit; water-skiing permitted outside limit; all craft must show insurance certificate before launching
Facilities:	parking for car and trailer (c), boat park (c), toilets
Dues:	none
Charge:	none
Directions:	from Kings Lynn take A149 north: turn off and follow signs
Waters accessed:	The Wash and North Sea

Kings Lynn - Common Staithe Quay

Tel: (01485) 535150 (Resort Manager)

Type:	concrete slipway
Suits:	all craft
Availability:	approx. 2 hours either side HW
Restrictions:	at LW thick mud is exposed
Facilities:	fuel, parking for car and trailer (c), toilets on site, chandlery nearby
Dues:	none
Charge:	approx. £15
Directions:	follow A10 north to Kings Lynn or A47 north west from Norwich
Waters accessed:	River Great Ouse and The Wash

Barton Turf - Cox Bros. Boatyard, Staithe Road
Tel: (01692) 536206

Type:	shallow wooden ramp
Suits:	sailing craft up to 600kg weight
Availability:	during working hours by prior arrangement
Restrictions:	4 and 5 mph speed limits: water-skiing prohibited
Facilities:	parking for car and trailer, toilets, outboard repairs, boat repairs and moorings all on site
Dues:	Broads Authority licence required
Charge:	approx. £5
Directions:	from Wroxham, go north towards Stalham, turning right to Barton Turf and following signs to river
Waters accessed:	Barton Broad and Norfolk Broads

Beccles - Beccles Yacht Station
Tel: (01502) 712225

Type:	concrete slipway
Suits:	all craft up to 20'/6.1m LOA
Availability:	approx. 3 hours either side HW
Restrictions:	4 mph speed limit
Facilities:	parking for car and trailer nearby, toilets
Dues:	Broads Authority licence required
Charge:	none
Directions:	follow A146 Beccles by-pass and signs to 'Quay'
Waters accessed:	River Waveney and Norfolk Broads

Beccles - Aston Boats, Bridge Wharf
Tel: (01502) 713960

Type:	concrete ramp
Suits:	all craft except pwc
Availability:	approx. 4 hours either side HW 0800-1700 by prior arrangement
Restrictions:	4 mph speed limit: pwc prohibited, water-skiing permitted in designated areas only
Facilities:	diesel, parking for car and trailer (c) and toilets on site, outboard repairs nearby
Dues:	Broads Authority licence required
Charge:	approx. £7
Directions:	from town centre, take old road to Norwich, crossing over river bridge: site is down drive 200m on right
Waters accessed:	River Waveney and Norfolk Broads

Beccles - H E Hipperson, Gillingham Dam
Tel: (01502) 712166

Type:	concrete slipway
Suits:	dinghies and small powered craft
Availability:	approx.1/2 hour either side HW by prior arrangement only

Restrictions:	4 mph speed limit: water-skiing permitted in designated areas with special licence
Facilities:	diesel on site, petrol from local garage, parking for car and trailer (c), toilets on site, outboard repairs nearby; caravan club site
Dues:	Broads Authority licence required
Charge:	approx. £4
Directions:	from Norwich follow A146 southeast to outskirts of Beccles; at roundabout take 2nd exit signposted Beccles and after 400m turn right through Gillingham: site is on left before river bridge
Waters accessed:	River Waveney

Beccles - Waveney Valley Boats, Puddingmoor

Tel: (01502) 712538

Type:	steel ramp
Suits:	dinghies and small powered craft up to 20'/6.1m LOA
Availability:	all states of tide 0900-1700 weekdays, 1100-1700 weekends by prior arrangement only
Restrictions:	4,5 and 7 mph speed limits: water-skiing permitted in designated areas only
Facilities:	diesel on site, petrol in town, parking for car and trailer (c), toilets, outboard repairs, chandlery and crane all on site
Dues:	Broads Authority licence required
Charge:	approx. £13; £30 with yard assistance
Directions:	from Bungay take A144 turning left onto B1062; at approach to town turn left into Puddingmoor: site is on left at town end of road
Waters accessed:	River Waveney and Norfolk Broads

Brundall - Brundall Bay Marina, Riverside Estate

Tel: (01603) 716606

Type:	concrete slipway
Suits:	sailing and small powered craft
Availability:	0830-1730 mon-fri: 0900-1500 sat and 1000-1400 sun by prior arrangement
Restrictions:	5 mph speed limit: ski-boats and pwc prohibited from site, parking of trailers by arrangement only; locked barrier outside hours
Facilities:	diesel on site, petrol nearby, parking for car (c) and trailer (c) by arrangement, toilets, outboard repairs on site, chandlery nearby
Dues:	Broads Authority licence required
Charge:	approx. £7.50
Directions:	from Norwich take A47 east towards Gt Yarmouth; at 1st roundabout take last exit signposted Brundall and turn right at Barclays Bank
Waters accessed:	River Yare and Norfolk Broads

Brundall - Bell Boats Ltd

Tel: (01603) 713109

Type:	launching by crane only
Suits:	craft up to 35 tons
Availability:	all states of tide during working hours
Restrictions:	speed limit
Facilities:	moorings, storage, boat repairs and servicing
Dues:	Broads Authority licence required
Charge:	approx. £42 + vat up to 20'/6.1m LOA, thereafter at £7 per metre
Directions:	from Norwich take A47 east towards Gt Yarmouth; at 1st roundabout take last exit signposted Brundall
Waters accessed:	River Yare and Norfolk Broads

Brundall - Harbour Cruisers, Riverside Estate

Tel: (01603) 712146

Type:	concrete slipway
Suits:	all craft
Availability:	all states of tide during working hours
Restrictions:	speed limit: pwc prohibited; water-skiing in designated area with special licence; locked barrier opens 0700 daily and closes 1800 in winter and 2100 in summer
Facilities:	diesel on site, petrol nearby, parking for car and trailer (c) and toilets on site, chandlery nearby
Dues:	Broads Authority licence required
Charge:	approx. £5
Directions:	from Norwich take A47 east towards Gt Yarmouth; at 1st roundabout take last exit signposted Brundall and turn right after 1 mile into Station Rd; site is half a mile on left
Waters accessed:	River Yare

Buckenham Ferry - Paul Wright Mouldings Ltd

Tel: (01508) 480218

Type:	metal mesh over gravel
Suits:	all craft up to 25'/7.6m LOA
Availability:	all states of tide during working hours
Restrictions:	speed limit: water-skiing permitted in designated areas with special licence
Facilities:	parking for car and trailer nearby (c), toilets nearby, fibreglass repairs on site, pub and restaurant adjacent to site
Dues:	Broads Authority licence required
Charge:	approx. £3
Directions:	from Norwich take A146, turning left at sign to Kirby Bedon, Rockland and Claxton: go through Claxton and after 1/2 mile look for sign to left to boatyard and river
Waters accessed:	River Yare and Norfolk Broads

Burgh Castle - Burgh Castle Marina, Butt Lane
Tel: (01493) 780331 Fax: 01493 780163

Type:	shallow concrete ramp
Suits:	all craft except windsurfers and pwc
Availability:	approx. 4 hours either side HW by prior arrangement to obtain weekly ticket and key to barrier
Restrictions:	6 mph speed limit: water-skiing permitted in designated area with special licence
Facilities:	diesel nearby, parking for car and trailer, toilets and showers, chandlery, static caravan site, touring caravans and tent site, pub, restaurant and shop all on site
Dues:	Broads Authority licence required
Charge:	approx. £21 + vat per week
Directions:	from Gt Yarmouth take A143 west following signs to Burgh Castle
Waters accessed:	River Waveney and South Broads

Burgh Castle - Goodchild Marine Services, Burgh Castle Yacht Station
Tel: (01493) 782301 Fax: 01493 782306

Type:	launching by 32 ton boat hoist
Suits:	larger craft
Availability:	all states of tide 0800-1800 by prior arrangement
Restrictions:	no speed limit on Breydon Water: water-skiing permitted with special licence
Facilities:	diesel, parking for car and trailer, toilets, chandlery, outboard repairs, rigging, pump-out and full boatyard services
Dues:	Broads Authority licence required
Charge:	approx. £30
Directions:	from Gt Yarmouth take A143 west, turning right approx. 2 miles after Gorleston roundabout and following signs to Burgh Castle and Belton: site entrance is 1/2 mile south of village
Waters accessed:	River Waveney and Breydon Water

Burgh St Peter - Waveney River Centre, Staithe Road
Tel: (01502) 677217/677343

Type:	medium concrete slipway
Suits:	dinghies and powered craft
Availability:	approx. 3-4 hours either side HW
Restrictions:	5 mph speed limit: water-skiing permitted in designated areas with special licence
Facilities:	fuel, parking for car and trailer, toilets and showers, chandlery, crane and boat lift, pub, shop and caravan site
Dues:	Broads Authority licence required
Charge:	approx. £5
Directions:	from Gt Yarmouth take A143 towards Beccles; after Haddiscoe turn left onto minor roads and follow signs
Waters accessed:	River Waveney

143

Hickling - Whispering Reeds Boats Ltd, Staithe Road
Tel: (01692) 598314

Type:	concrete slipway
Suits:	craft up to 21'/6.5m LOA except pwc
Availability:	0800-1700 mon-sat; Easter to end Oct 0900-1700 sun
Restrictions:	4-6 mph speed limit: water-skiing permitted in designated areas with special licence; locked barrier outside hours
Facilities:	fuel at Martham, parking for car and trailer, (c) for trailer if left more than 1 day, toilets and shower: chandlery and outboard repairs from Wroxham; Hickling Broad is the largest Broad and an important nature reserve - and famous for its sponge weed
Dues:	Broads Authority licence required (available here)
Charge:	approx. £8
Directions:	from Norwich take A1151 through Wroxham; at junction with A149 turn right through Stalham and after approx. 2½ miles turn left to Hickling; at 'T' junction turn left and at next crossroads right; site is past Pleasure Boat Inn
Waters accessed:	Hickling Broad

Horning - next The Swan Inn, The Street
Tel: (01692) 630434 (Ralph's Newsagents)

Type:	concrete slipway
Suits:	small craft
Availability:	at all times
Restrictions:	speed limit: water-skiing permitted in designated area with special licence; access is via locked barrier - key from Ralph's Newsagents in Lower Street
Facilities:	fuel in village, limited parking for car and trailer, toilets nearby
Dues:	Broads Authority licence required
Charge:	approx. £5 + £5 deposit (refundable) for key
Directions:	from Norwich take A1151 to Wroxham, turning right onto A1062 and right again into Horning village
Waters accessed:	River Bure and South Broads

Loddon - Mistral Craft, Bridge Street
Tel: (01508) 520438

Type:	steep concrete ramp (1:8.5)
Suits:	all craft except windsurfers
Availability:	approx. 3 hours either side HW by prior arrangement
Restrictions:	3 mph speed limit: no pwc, water-skiing or windsurfing
Facilities:	fuel nearby, parking for car and trailer on site (c), toilets nearby
Dues:	Broads Authority licence required
Charge:	approx. £10

| Directions: | from Norwich southern by-pass take A146 to Lowestoft and after 8 miles take road signposted to Loddon: site is in main street |
| Waters accessed: | Norfolk Broads |

Martham - Martham Boat Building Co, Riverside, Cess Road
Tel: (01493) 740249

Type:	concrete slipway
Suits:	dinghies, trailer-sailers and small powered craft
Availability:	0800-1630
Restrictions:	4 mph speed limit: no windsurfing, pwc or water-skiing allowed
Facilities:	fuel, parking for car and trailer (c), toilets, pump-out, showers
Dues:	Broads Authority licence required
Charge:	approx. £9
Directions:	from Gt Yarmouth take A149 north; turn right onto B1152 to Martham
Waters accessed:	River Thurne and Norfolk Broads

Oulton Broad - Water Sports Centre, St Nicholas Everitt Park
Tel: (01502) 587163

Type:	concrete slipway
Suits:	all craft except pwc
Availability:	approx. 3 hours either side HW by prior arrangement
Restrictions:	4 knot speed limit: pwc and water-skiing prohibited; site enclosure locked when not in use
Facilities:	parking for car and trailer (c) and chandlery nearby, toilets on site
Dues:	Broads Authority licence required
Charge:	none
Directions:	from Lowestoft follow A146; site is south of road bridge
Waters accessed:	Oulton Broad, Norfolk Broads and North Sea

Oulton Broad - Pegasus Yachts, Caldecott Road
Tel: (01502) 585631

Type:	shallow concrete ramp
Suits:	all craft except pwc and windsurfers
Availability:	approx. 2 hours either side HW by prior arrangement
Restrictions:	6 mph speed limit: pwc and water-skiing prohibited
Facilities:	fuel nearby, parking for car and trailer, outboard repairs, crane and tractor: toilets and chandlery nearby
Dues:	Broads Authority licence required
Charge:	approx. £5 ; £10 for powered craft
Directions:	site is on north side of Oulton Broad
Waters accessed:	Oulton Broad, Norfolk Broads and North Sea

Oulton Broad - The Commodore Pub

Tel: (01502) 565955

Type:	concrete slipway
Suits:	small craft
Availability:	at all times by arrangement with pub
Restrictions:	6 mph speed limit; water-skiing prohibited
Facilities:	fuel nearby, parking for car and trailer (c), chandlery nearby, toilets
Dues:	Broads Authority licence required
Charge:	none
Directions:	take A146 towards Beccles: pub is on north side of bridge
Waters accessed:	Oulton Broad

Oulton Broad - Colmans Land Slipway, Bridge Road

Type:	concrete slipway
Suits:	small craft
Availability:	at all times
Restrictions:	speed limit: water-skiing prohibited
Facilities:	fuel, parking for car and trailer (c), toilets and chandlers nearby
Dues:	Broads Authority licence required
Charge:	none
Directions:	from Lowestoft take A146 towards Beccles: site is south of bridge and Nicholas Everitt Park on right
Waters accessed:	Oulton Broad, Norfolk Broads and North Sea

Reedham Ferry - Reedham Ferry Inn, Ferry Road

Tel: (01493) 700429 (Mr Archer)

Type:	shallow concrete ramp to river with drop
Suits:	all craft
Availability:	during daylight hours
Restrictions:	5 mph speed limit: water-skiing permitted in designated area nearby; keep clear of chain ferry and beware of deceptive tidal flow; private slipway - permission of owner always required
Facilities:	fuel nearby, parking for car and trailer, toilets, pub and restaurant, chandlery and outboard repairs nearby
Dues:	Broads Authority licence required
Charge:	approx. £5 inc. parking
Directions:	from Norwich take A47 towards Gt Yarmouth; turn right onto B1140 south at Damgate
Waters accessed:	River Yare and Norfolk Broads

Repps - Repps Staithe

Type:	concrete slipway
Suits:	craft up to 16'/4.9m LOA
Availability:	all states of tide
Restrictions:	speed limit
Facilities:	limited parking for car and trailer (c)

Dues:	Broads Authority licence required
Charge:	none
Directions:	take A149 north, turning left onto minor road to Repps
Waters accessed:	River Thurne and Norfolk Broads

St Olaves - next Bridge, Beccles Road

Tel: (01493) 488230 (Bridge Stores - Mrs M.C.Miller)

Type:	shallow concrete ramp
Suits:	small craft only
Availability:	at all times by prior arrangement
Restrictions:	speed limit: locked access, obtain key from Bridge Stores
Facilities:	fuel and parking for car and trailer nearby, shop, pub
Dues:	Broads Authority licence required
Charge:	approx. £5
Directions:	from Gt Yarmouth take A143 towards Beccles: site is by bridge opposite Bell Inn
Waters accessed:	River Waveney

Stalham - Richardsons Boatyard

Tel: (01692) 581081

Type:	shallow concrete ramp
Suits:	all craft up to 40'/12m LOA
Availability:	all times during working hours mon- fri, 0900-1230 on sun
Restrictions:	4 mph speed limit: water-skiing and pwc prohibited
Facilities:	diesel on site, parking for car and trailer (c), toilets and showers, crane, repairs and overhauls on site; chandlery and outboard repairs nearby
Dues:	Broads Authority licence required
Charge:	approx. £10
Directions:	from Norwich take A1151 and turn left onto A149 to Stalham
Waters accessed:	River Ant and Norfolk Broads

Stalham - Stalham Yacht Services Ltd, The Staithe

Tel: (01692) 580288 Fax: (01692) 582636

Type:	crane by arrangemant
Suits:	larger craft
Availability:	0800-1700 mon-fri; sat & sun by arrangement
Restrictions:	4-6 mph speed limit: pwc and water-skiing prohibited
Facilities:	diesel, parking for car and trailer (c), toilets and boatyard on site
Dues:	Broads Authority licence required
Charge:	approx. £20
Directions:	from Norwich take A1151 and turn left onto A149 to Stalham following signs to Staithe
Waters accessed:	River Ant and Norfolk Broads

Thorpe - Griffin Marine, 10 Griffin Lane
Tel: (01603) 433253

Type:	concrete slipway into 4'/1.2m water
Suits:	all craft up to 20'/6.1m LOA
Availability:	at all times
Restrictions:	3-6 mph speed limits: pwc prohibited; water-skiing permitted in designated area with special licence; access to main river is under railway bridge with 6'/1.83m headroom
Facilities:	parking for car and trailer (c if more than 1 day), toilets, chandlery, outboard repairs, full engineering and boatyard facilties, fishing tackle and bait all on site
Dues:	Broads Authority licence required
Charge:	approx. £5
Directions:	take Norwich take A47 (southern by-pass) turning off at Norwich East/Thorpe
Waters accessed:	River Yare and Norfolk Broads

Wroxham - Landamores Boatyard, Marsh Rd, Hoveton
Tel: (01603) 782212

Type:	concrete slipway
Suits:	all craft with up to 2'/0.6m draught on trailer
Availability:	at all times: prior arrangement preferred
Restrictions:	4/5 mph speed limit: pwc, windsurfing and water-skiing prohibited; access may be restricted by parked cars and locked barrier
Facilities:	fuel nearby, parking for car and trailer (c), toilets, chandlery, crane and boatyard facilities on site, outboard repairs nearby
Dues:	Broads Authority licence required
Charge:	approx. £6
Directions:	from Norwich take A1151, turning right at crossroads after Wroxham Bridge into Church Rd and right again into Marsh Rd
Waters accessed:	River Bure

Wroxham - Moore & Co, Staitheway Road
Tel: (01603) 783311

Type:	concrete slipway
Suits:	all craft up to 35'/10.7m LOA
Availability:	at all times during working hours
Restrictions:	5 mph speed limit: access to site is via locked barrier
Facilities:	diesel on site, petrol nearby, parking for car and trailer (c), toilets and Leisure Centre on site; chandlery and outboard repairs nearby
Dues:	Broads Authority licence required
Charge:	approx. £24
Directions:	from Norwich take A1151 to Wroxham; in Wroxham, turn right into the Avenues and 1st left into Staitheway Rd; site is at end of road
Waters accessed:	River Bure and Norfolk Broads

LAKE SITES

Milton Keynes - Willen Lake - Watersports, Willen Lake, Brickhill Street
Tel: (01908) 670197

Type:	two shallow concrete ramps
Suits:sailing	dinghies, windsurfers and canoes up to 18'/5.5m LOA
Availability:	0900 - ½ hour before dusk mon-fri: 0900-1830 weekends
Restrictions:	powered craft prohibited
Facilities:	petrol nearby, parking for car and trailer, toilets, chandlery, hotel and bar facilities all on site
Dues:	no additional fee charged
Charge:	approx.£10-12
Directions:	leave M1 at junction 14 and take A509 west for approx. 2 miles
Waters accessed:	Willen Lake

Grafham Water - Grafham Water S.C.
Tel: (01480) 810478

Type:	concrete slipway
Suits:	sailing dinghies, trailer-sailers and windsurfers
Availability:	0930-1 hour before sunset
Restrictions:	no powered craft
Facilities:	parking for car and trailer, toilets, chandlery, windsurfing shop and RYA courses in windsurfing, dinghy and catamaran sailing
Dues:	none
Charge:	approx.£4.50 per craft plus £4.50 per person, weekdays; £7.50 per craft and £7.50 per person, sun
Directions:	from A1 take B661 at Buckden roundabout, continue for approx. 2 miles to village of Perry and turn right opposite ' Wheatsheaf' pub: site is at end of road
Waters accessed:	Grafham Water

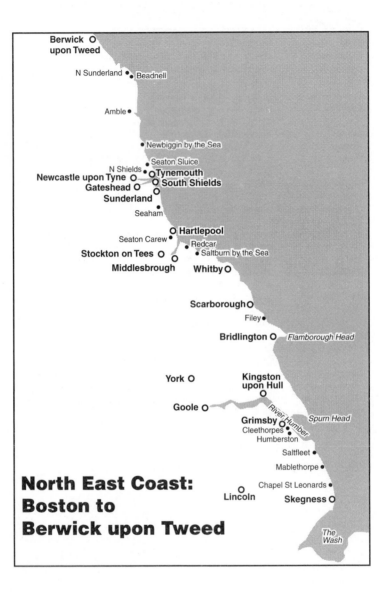

Berwick
upon Tweed O

N Sunderland • • Beadnell

Amble •

• Newbiggin by the Sea

• Seaton Sluice
N Shields • O Tynemouth
Newcastle upon Tyne O O South Shields
Gateshead O
Sunderland •
Seaham •

Seaton Carew • O Hartlepool
• Redcar
Stockton on Tees O • Saltburn by the Sea
Middlesbrough O Whitby O

Scarborough O
Filey •

Bridlington O Flamborough Head

York O Kingston
upon Hull
O

Goole O
Grimsby O River Humber Spurn Head
Cleethorpes •
Humberston •

Saltfleet •

Mablethorpe •

Chapel St Leonards •
Lincoln O Skegness O

North East Coast:
Boston to
Berwick upon Tweed

The
Wash

Skegness - Princes Parade
Tel: (01754) 768854 (T.K.Wallis, Chairman - Skegness Boating Club)

Type:	tractor-assisted launching over sand
Suits:	craft up to 20'/6.1m LOA
Availability:	all states of tide with prior permission
Restrictions:	site is controlled by Skegness Boating Club: keys to locked barrier available to members only; all craft must carry safety equipment
Facilities:	parking for car and trailer on site, toilets nearby, boat and trailer storage on site
Dues:	none
Charge:	annual membership available to casual visitors (subject to committee approval)
Directions:	from town centre, turn south along seafront and left into Princes Parade car park: club premises are on right
Waters accessed:	The Wash and North Sea

Skegness - Gibraltar Point
Tel: (01754) 890209 (Mr J.Elkins, Secretary - Skegness Yacht Club)

Type:	concrete slipway
Suits:	dinghies and trailer-sailers
Availability:	approx. 1 hour either side HW with prior permission
Restrictions	4 knot speed limit; powercraft and pwc prohibited; site is controlled by Skegness Y.C. - contact Secretary for permission and advice
Facilities:	toilets and parking for car and trailer in nearby nature reserve car park (c)
Dues:	none
Charge:	approx. £2
Directions:	follow minor road approx. 3 miles south from town centre: site is at entrance to Wainfleet Creek on Lincolnshire Trust Nature Reserve
Waters accessed:	The Wash and North Sea

Skegness - Jacksons Corner, Ingoldmells
Tel: (01509) 880526 (Mr Ballard - Skegness Water Sports Club)

Type:	tractor-assisted launching over sand from shallow concrete ramp
Suits:	small sailing and powered craft up to 22'/6.7m LOA
Availability:	0900-1900 at weekends: weekdays by prior arrangement only
Restrictions:	site is controlled by Skegness Water Sports Club - contact Secretary; all boats launched must have insurance; all craft to operate 200m from shore
Facilities:	parking for car and trailer, toilets, changing rooms and storage
Dues:	none
Charge:	approx. £10

Directions:	follow A52 north from Skegness to Mablethorpe, turning at side of Butlin's Funcoast Camp and following signs to sea
Waters accessed:	North Sea

Chapel St Leonards - Beach

Type:	pullover onto sand to north of village
Suits:	light craft which can be manhandled; tractor assistance may be available from local fishermen
Availability:	all states of tide over beach
Restrictions:	motor vehicles are not allowed on the central pullover
Facilities:	parking for car and trailer (c), toilets
Dues:	none
Charge:	none, but may be charge for tractor
Directions:	follow A52 and minor roads approx 6 miles north from Skegness
Waters accessed:	North Sea

Sandilands - Sea Lane Pullover

Type:	pullover onto sandy beach
Suits:	light craft which can be manhandled; tractor assistance may be available from local fishermen
Availability:	all states of tide
Restrictions:	none
Facilities:	parking for car and trailer (c), toilets, water-skiing and pwc permitted
Dues:	none
Charge:	none, but may be charge for tractor
Directions:	follow A52 and minor roads north from Skegness
Waters accessed:	North Sea

Sutton-on-Sea - Church Lane Pullover

Type:	pullover onto sandy beach
Suits:	light craft which can be manhandled over beach
Availability:	all states of tide over beach
Restrictions:	motor vehicles are not allowed on the pullover
Facilities:	parking for car and trailer in village (1/4 mile), toilets and cafe on site; pubs approx. 200m
Dues:	none
Charge:	none
Directions:	follow A52 north from Skegness: site is approx. 3 miles south of Mablethorpe
Waters accessed:	North Sea

Mablethorpe - Seaholme Road Pullover

Type:	pullover onto sandy beach
Suits:	light craft which can be manhandled
Availability:	all states of tide
Restrictions:	water-skiing and pwc prohibited
Facilities:	parking for car and trailer (c), toilets, cafe and pub on site

Dues: none
Charge: none
Directions: follow A52 north from Skegness
Waters accessed: North Sea

Saltfleet - Saltfleet Haven

Tel: (01507) 338542 (Mr Carter - Saltfleet Haven Boat Club)

Type:	stone slipway
Suits:	craft up to 25'/7.6m LOA
Availability:	approx. 2 hours either side HW
Restrictions:	site is controlled by Saltfleet Haven Boat Club: bar with narrow gap at entrance to Haven; site is dangerous in onshore winds; water-skiing prohibited in Haven
Facilities:	parking for car and trailer
Dues:	none
Charge:	yes
Directions:	follow A1031 south from Cleethorpes
Waters accessed:	North Sea

Humberston - Humber Mouth Yacht Club

Tel: (01472) 329788 (Mr J Clegg - Hon. Secretary)

Type:	concrete slipway onto beach
Suits:	all craft
Availability:	approx. 1½ hours either side HW with prior permission
Restrictions:	8 knot speed limit inshore: water-skiing and pwc permitted offshore
Facilities:	parking for car and trailer, toilets, tractor assistance, chandlery, outboard repairs and diving supplies all available, clubhouse for use of members of RYA affiliated clubs, shops (in season) in nearby caravan park
Dues:	none
Charge:	none, but may be for tractor assistance
Directions:	follow A18 and signed route to holiday attractions: site is at end of metalled track through Thorpe Park Holiday Camp
Waters accessed:	Tetney Haven, Humber Estuary and North Sea

Cleethorpes - Pier Slipway

Tel: (01472) 698828 (Beach Safety Officer)

Type:	concrete slipway onto shingle
Suits:	all craft with up to 3'/1m draught
Availability:	approx. 2 hours either side HW
Restrictions:	8 knot speed limit within 200m of shore: water-skiing permitted in designated area with access channel; no parking on or obstruction of slipway which must be kept clear for lifeboat
Facilities:	fuel nearby, parking for car and trailer (c), toilets, chandlery
Dues:	none
Charge:	none

| Directions: | follow A46 from Lincoln or M180/A180: site is next to Pier at end of Sea Road |
| Waters accessed: | Humber Estuary and North Sea |

Cleethorpes - Brighton Street Slipway
Tel: (01472) 698828 (Beach Safety Officer)

Type:	cobbles and concrete slipway
Suits:	small craft which can be manhandled: larger craft should use Pier Slipway
Availability:	approx. 2 hours either side HW
Restrictions:	8 knot speed limit within 200m of shore: water-skiing in designated area with access channel; no parking on or obstruction of slipway which must be kept clear for lifeboat
Facilities:	fuel, parking for car and trailer (c), toilets and chandlery nearby
Dues:	none
Charge:	none
Directions:	follow A46 from Lincoln or M180/A180: site is on seafront opposite Brighton Street
Waters accessed:	Humber Estuary and North Sea

Cleethorpes - Wonderland Slipway
Tel: (01472) 698828 (Beach Safety Officer)

Type:	launching across beach by 4-wheel drive vehicles only
Suits:	small craft which can be manhandled: larger craft should use Pier Slipway
Availability:	at all states of tide across beach
Restrictions:	8 knot speed limit within 200m of shore: water-skiing permitted in designated area with access channel; no parking on beach; 4-wheel drive vehicle essential to cross beach
Facilities:	fuel, parking for car and trailer (c), toilets and chandlery nearby
Dues:	none
Charge:	none
Directions:	follow A46 from Lincoln or M180/A180 to Cleethorpes then go down Sea Road and turn left onto the Promenade and site is at north end
Waters accessed:	Humber Estuary and North Sea

Goole - Goole Boathouse, Dutch Riverside
Tel: (01405) 763985

Type:	concrete ramp (1:8)
Suits:	all craft except pwc and windsurfers
Availability:	during working hours or by prior arrangement if outside hours
Restrictions:	6 mph speed limit on Aire and Calder Canal
Facilities:	diesel on site, petrol nearby, parking for car and trailer(c), toilets and chandlery on site
Dues:	BW licence required for canal

Charge:	approx. £5
Directions:	from junction 36 on M62, head into Goole: turn right at first traffic lights then follow signs to 'Waterways Museum'
Waters accessed:	Aire & Calder Canal, Rivers Ouse and Trent and Humber Estuary

Kingston-upon-Hull (River Humber) - Hessle Beach

Tel: (01482) 326338 (Harbour Master)

Type:	stone and shingle foreshore
Suits:	light craft which can be manhandled
Availability:	approx. 3 hours either side HW
Restrictions:	none
Facilities:	parking for car and trailer, local rescue group operates nearby
Dues:	none
Charge:	none
Directions:	leave M180 at junction 5 taking A15 over Humber Bridge: site is just downstream of bridge
Waters accessed:	River Humber and North Sea

Kingston-upon-Hull (River Humber) - Horsewash Slope, Victoria Pier

Tel: (01482) 613385 (Harbour Master)

Type:	stone slope
Suits:	light craft which can be manhandled
Availability:	approx. 2 hours either side HW by prior arrangement with Harbour Master
Restrictions	narrow access road on a bend and height restriction of approx. 12'/3.6m: site may be obstructed by shipping lying alongside
Facilities:	parking for car but not trailer nearby
Dues:	none
Charge:	none
Directions:	leave M62 at Jct 8 following A63: turn right at cross-roads before Myton Bridge and proceed to pier (approx. 200m); site is just east of Hull Marina
Waters accessed:	River Humber and North Sea

Bridlington - Belvedere Launch Site, Belvedere Parade

Tel: (01262) 673761/678255

Type:	concrete slipway onto hard sand
Suits:	all craft up to 20'/6.1m LOA
Availability:	0800 to 1 hour before sunset 1st Apr-31st Oct: by appointment only in Apr and Oct
Restrictions:	8 knot speed limit within 300m of LWS mark: water-skiing permitted outside limit; all boats are inspected prior to launch and local regulations concerning insurance and safety equipment must be complied with; access to site is via a locked barrier

Facilities:	fuel from garage, parking for car and trailer, toilets, tractor assistance available, secure boat park; chandlery, diving supplies and outboard repairs all available nearby
Dues:	none
Charge:	approx. £6
Directions:	follow A166 from York or A165 from Hull
Waters accessed:	North Sea

Bridlington - South Landing, Flamborough

Tel: (01262) 678255

Type:	tarmac slipway onto stone and sand
Suits:	all craft up to 20'/6.1m LOA: tractor assistance available
Availability:	0800 to 1 hour before sunset 1st Apr-31st Oct
Restrictions:	8 knot speed limit within 300m of LWS mark: water-skiing permitted offshore; trailers must be parked in car park at top of slipway; slip is used by Flamborough RNLI Lifeboat and must be kept clear at all times; all boats are inspected prior to launch and local regulations concerning insurance and safety equipment must be complied with
Facilities:	fuel from village, parking for car and trailer nearby, toilets (200m), chandlery, diving supplies and outboard repairs all in town
Dues:	none
Charge:	approx. £6 (pay in machine at top of slipway)
Directions:	follow A166 from York or A165 from Hull north through Bridlington; turning east onto B1255 to Flamborough: site is to south of village
Waters accessed:	North Sea

Filey - Filey Coble Landing

Tel: (01723) 373530 (Harbour Dept.)

Type:	shallow slipway of concrete and stone setts onto sand; at certain times there may be a small drop at end of slipway
Suits:	sailing craft and small powered craft: no pwc
Availability:	all states of tide (approx. 2 hours either side HW for larger craft)
Restrictions:	speed limit within 200m of shore: water-skiing permitted outside this area; boats with engine capacity over 20hp prohibited
Facilities:	parking for car nearby (c) and trailer can be left on sand with permission from Harbour Master/Beach Attendant (c), toilets nearby
Dues:	none
Charge:	approx. £5.80
Directions:	follow A64 and A1039 from York: site is at north end of sea front
Waters accessed:	North Sea

Scarborough Harbour - Golden Ball Slipway
Tel: (01723) 373877 (Harbour Master)

Type:	shallow concrete ramp with stone setts
Suits:	all craft except pwc and windsurfers
Availability:	approx. 3 hours either side HW
Restrictions:	low speed in harbour: slipway has locked barrier - contact duty watchkeeper; trailers must be removed from slipway
Facilities:	diesel nearby, parking for car and trailer nearby (c), toilets, chandlery and outboard repairs nearby
Dues:	approx £7.20 per day (£103 p.a.)
Charge:	no additional fee
Directions:	follow A64 from York to Scarborough: site is off Harbour Side Rd
Waters accessed:	North Sea

Whitby - Whitby Marina, off Langbourne Road
Tel: (01947) 600165 (Harbour Dept.)

Type:	shallow concrete ramp
Suits:	all craft
Availability:	approx. 4 hours either side of HW
Restrictions:	speed limit: water-skiing prohibited in harbour
Facilities:	fuel nearby, parking for car and trailer on site (c), toilets and chandlery on site, diving supplies and outboard repairs nearby
Dues:	approx £8.50
Charge:	no additional fee
Directions:	follow A171 east from Middlesbrough or A64/A169 from York: turn right in centre of town past Co-op supermarket
Waters accessed:	River Esk and North Sea

Skinningrove

Type:	launching over shingle foreshore
Suits:	small craft which can be manhandled
Availability:	approx. 2/3 hours either side of HW
Restrictions:	access is via narrow road
Facilities:	limited parking for car and trailer on site
Dues:	none
Charge:	none
Directions:	follow A174 from Middlesbrough or Whitby
Waters accessed:	North Sea

Saltburn-by-the-Sea - Seafront

Type:	launching over shingle and firm sand
Suits:	dinghies only
Availability:	approx. 2/3 hours either side HW
Restrictions:	exposed sea conditions in onshore winds
Facilities:	fuel in village, parking for car and trailer on site (c), toilets

Dues:	none
Charge:	none
Directions:	follow A174 from Whitby or Middlesbrough: site is near pier
Waters accessed:	North Sea

Redcar - Seafront

Type:	three wide concrete slipways onto firm sand
Suits:	small craft
Availability:	all states of tide but best 2-3 hours either side HW
Restrictions:	exposed conditions in onshore winds, local knowledge is essential
Facilities:	fuel in town, parking for car and trailer (c), toilets
Dues:	none
Charge:	none
Directions:	follow A1085 from Middlesbrough
Waters accessed:	North Sea

Redcar (River Tees) - South Gare Marine Club, South Gare
Tel: (01642) 491039 or 494099 (evenings) (Secretary R. Finch)

Type:	concrete slipway with winch and snatch block available
Suits:	all craft
Availability:	all times except 1 hour either side LWS, by prior arrangement
Restrictions:	water-skiing in designated areas: tides may be strong at river mouth; all craft must register with the Harbour Office, Tees Dock Tel: (01642) 277205; access to site is via private road which may be shut at odd times and by locked barrier at entrance to club
Facilities:	parking for car and trailer (c), toilets
Dues:	registration fee
Charge:	yes
Directions:	follow A1085 from Middlesbrough to Coatham taking Sea Front Road at traffic lights by Cowies Garage and turning left at roundabout: club will be seen on left after about 3 miles; access is via single track private road with passing places
Waters accessed:	River Tees and North Sea

Thornaby (River Tees) - Tees Barrage, Navigation Way
Tel: (01642) 633273 - VHF Ch 37 (Tees Barrage Ltd.)

Type:	shallow concrete slipway
Suits:	all craft
Availability:	at all times
Restrictions:	5 mph speed limit on river: water-skiing and pwc permitted for club members only in designated areas; all powered craft must be registered with Tees Barrage Ltd. and have proof of 3rd party liability insurance; craft intending to enter the tidal waters downstream of the lock must register with the Tees Harbour Office Tel: (01642) 277205

Facilities:	parking for car and trailer on site, boat lift up to 12 tonne @ £50
Dues:	registration fee
Charge:	approx. £10
Directions:	site is signposted off the A66 west of the A19
Waters accessed:	non-tidal River Tees or lock through to tidal river and North Sea

Stockton-on-Tees (River Tees) - Corporation Quay, Riverside Rd
Tel: (01642) 633273 - VHF Ch 37 (Tees Barrage Ltd.)

Type:	concrete slipway
Suits:	all craft up to 20'/6.1m LOA approx.
Availability:	at all times
Restrictions:	5 mph speed limit on river: water-skiing and pwc permitted for club members only in designated areas; all powered craft must be registered with Tees Barrage Ltd. and have proof of 3rd party liability insurance; all users must sign a disclaimer from Stockton B.C.; craft intending to enter the tidal waters downstream of the lock must register with the Tees Harbour Office Tel: (01642) 277205
Facilities:	petrol nearby, parking for car and trailer
Dues:	registration fee
Charge:	none
Directions:	follow A1(M) north turning off onto A66 and following signs to Stockton: access is via car park in Riverside Road
Waters accessed:	non-tidal River Tees or lock through to tidal river and North Sea

Seaton Carew - Seafront
Tel: (01429) 221824 (Foreshore Officer - Hartlepool Borough Council)

Type:	concrete slipway with slope onto soft sand
Suits:	small powered craft
Availability:	approx. 4 hours either side HW by prior arrangement
Restrictions:	all craft must keep clear of shipping channels; exposed conditions in onshore winds; local knowledge is necessary; vehicles allowed on beach only with permission
Facilities:	parking for car and trailer (c)
Dues:	none
Charge:	none
Directions:	follow A19 from Teesside, then A689 and B1276 to seafront
Waters accessed:	North Sea

Hartlepool - Hartlepool Marina
Tel: (01429) 865744 VHF Ch 37/80 (Marina Office)

Type:	concrete slipway onto shingle and hard sand
Suits:	all craft except pwc and windsurfers
Availability:	approx. 3 hours either side HW; access available via marina lock office
Restrictions:	4 knot speed limit: no mooring or anchoring in West Harbour
Facilities:	petrol nearby, diesel, parking for car and trailer, toilets and showers, chandlery, outboard repairs and overnight berths all on site, diving supplies nearby; 24 hour lock access
Dues:	none
Charge:	none
Directions:	follow A19 from Teesside, then A172 , turning right at roundabout, going straight across 4 sets of traffic lights then right at 'T' junction: site is on left behind cabins alongside inner North Pier
Waters accessed:	Hartlepool Bay and North Sea

Hartlepool - Tees Sailing Club, West Harbour
Tel: (01429) 265400

Type:	concrete slipway
Suits:	all craft up to 5 tons
Availability:	approx. 4 hours either side HW, Wed pm, all day Sat and Sun or by prior arrangement
Restrictions:	4 knot speed limit in harbour; no mooring or anchoring permitted in West Harbour
Facilities:	diesel from marina, parking for car and trailer and toilets on site; chandlery, outboard repairs, diving supplies, overnight berths and showers in marina; 24 hour lock access
Dues:	none
Charge:	approx. £5
Directions:	follow A19 then A689 to town centre, turning right near 'The Mail' office down Church St: turn left at traffic lights over level crossing and proceed until S.C. on right
Waters accessed:	Hartlepool Bay and North Sea

Seaham Harbour - Harbour Slipway, North Dock
Tel: (0191) 5813246 (Harbour Office)

Type:	steep concrete slipway
Suits:	all craft up to 24'/7.3m LOA and 5'/1.5m draught except pwc
Availability:	approx. 2 hours either side HW
Restrictions:	5 knot speed limit: water-skiing and pwc prohibited; security must be advised of intention to launch on arrival at site
Facilities:	fuel nearby, parking for car and trailer nearby

Dues:	none
Charge:	approx. £6
Directions:	follow A19 north from Middlesbrough, turning onto B1285; site is adjacent to centre of Seaham
Waters accessed:	North Sea

Sunderland (River Wear) - Claxhaugh Rock

Tel: (0191) 5532100 (Port of Sunderland)

Type:	shallow concrete slipway
Suits:	all craft up to 20'/6.1m LOA except pwc and wind-surfers
Availability:	approx. 3 hours either side HW
Restrictions:	6 knot speed limit: water-skiing permitted in designated area only; pwc prohibited
Facilities:	parking for car and trailer on site
Dues:	approx. £6 + vat; (£32.50 + vat p.a.)
Charge:	no additional fee
Directions:	from A19 turn onto A183 at sign 'Sunderland South': turn left at first roundabout, left at next roundabout and ask for directions when river is reached: site is 4 miles from river mouth
Waters accessed:	River Wear and North Sea

Roker - Inshore Lifeboat Slip, Marine Walk

Tel: (0191) 553 2100 (Port of Sunderland)

Type:	short shallow concrete ramp onto soft sandy beach
Suits:	small craft which can be manhandled
Availability:	all states of tide
Restrictions:	6 knot speed limit: water-skiing prohibited but pwc permitted outside piers; no motorised vehicles on beaches; Inshore Lifeboat launches from ramp which must be kept clear at all times; Inshore Superintendent's Office is on Marine Walk
Facilities:	fuel, parking for car and trailer, toilets and chandlery nearby; watersports centre for canoes, windsurfing etc. nearby
Dues:	approx. £6 (£32.50 + vat p.a.)
Charge:	none
Directions:	follow A183 north from town centre: where Harbour View joins Roker Terrace take Pier View Rd to Marine Walk: site is near North Pier
Waters accessed:	North Sea

Roker (River Wear) - Sunderland Marina

Tel: (0191) 5144721 (Marina Manager)

Type:	medium concrete ramp into river
Suits:	all craft
Availability:	all states of tide by prior arrangement
Restrictions:	6 knot speed limit in harbour and river: water-skiing permitted only in designated area; locked barrier to slipway

Facilities:	diesel on site, petrol nearby, parking for car and trailer, toilets and showers nearby; overnight berths in marina with 24 hour access
Dues:	none
Charge:	approx £80 p.a.
Directions:	from A1 take A690 and A19 north; turn right onto A1231 east to Roker following signs to seafront and 'National Glass Centre': site gives access to River Wear 10 mins from the open sea
Waters accessed:	River Wear and North Sea

South Shields - Groyne Launching Ramp, Little Haven Beach

Tel: Easter to Sept (0191) 4557411 or (0191) 4546612 all year

Type:	concrete slipway
Suits:	all craft
Availability:	all states of tide except 1 hour either side LWS with permit
Restrictions:	6 knot speed limit: no water-skiing or pwc in harbour; permit available from T.I.C., Sea Road or from Central Library, Prince George Sq; certificate of 3rd party insurance for £1,000,000 + is needed to obtain permit
Facilities:	fuel nearby, parking for car nearby and for trailer on site, toilets and diving supplies nearby
Dues:	none
Charge:	approx. £8.50 or £27.50 p.a. inc. parking
Directions:	follow A6115 south from Newcastle,or A1 then A194 to South Shields and follow signs to seafront
Waters accessed:	River Tyne and North Sea

Gateshead (River Tyne) - Friar's Goose Water Sports Club, Felling

Tel: (0191) 4692545 or 4692952 (eves)

Type:	concrete slipway
Suits:	all craft
Availability:	approx. 2-3 hours either side HW
Restrictions:	6 knot speed limit in river
Facilities:	fuel nearby, parking for car and trailer, toilets nearby, moorings
Dues:	none
Charge:	approx. £5
Directions:	follow A6127 from A1(M) into Gateshead: site is on south bank and access is via Green Lane
Waters accessed:	River Tyne and North Sea

Derwenthaugh (River Tyne) - Derwenthaugh Marina, Blaydon

Tel: (0191) 4140065 (Powerhouse Marine)

Type:	two medium concrete ramps
Suits:	craft up to 35'/10.7m LOA approx
Availability:	approx. 4½ hours either side HW
Restrictions:	6 knot speed limit upstream: fast water zone down-steam; all craft launching must have 3rd party insurance

Facilities:	fuel nearby, parking for car and trailer, toilets, showers and changing rooms, chandlery, outboard repairs and moorings
Dues:	none
Charge:	approx. £7
Directions:	from A1 follow signs to Blaydon (A 695) and look for blue building with 'ARCO': follow narrow road past this building to marina
Waters accessed:	River Tyne and North Sea

Newburn (River Tyne) - Tyne Riverside Country Park, Grange Road
Tel: (0191) 2640014 (Newburn Leisure Centre)

Type:	fairly steep concrete slipway
Suits:	small craft except pwc and windsurfers
Availability:	approx. 2½ hours either side HW for club members only
Restrictions:	6 mph speed limit: site has locked barrier; zoned areas for sailing, water-skiing etc but pwc prohibited; number of water-ski craft is restricted
Facilities:	fuel (½ mile), parking for car and trailer, toilets, changing facilities, refreshments; chandlery and outboard repairs nearby
Dues:	none
Charge:	approx. £6.50
Directions:	from A69 take the A6085 for Throckley / Newburn: turn off in Newburn into Grange Road and follow signs
Waters accessed:	River Tyne and North Sea

Hebburn (River Tyne) - Hebburn Marina Boat Club
Tel: (0191) 2640014 (Newburn Leisure Centre)

Type:	very steep concrete ramp
Suits:	small powered craft
Availability:	approx. 4 hours either side HW
Restrictions:	6 mph knot speed limit: no water-skiing
Facilities:	fuel and parking for car and trailer nearby
Dues:	none
Charge:	approx. £6.50
Directions:	from A69 take the A6085 for Throckley / Newburn turning off into Grange Road and following signs to 'Hebburn Riverside Park'
Waters accessed:	River Tyne and North Sea

North Shields (River Tyne) - Royal Quays Marina, Coble Dene Road
Tel: (0191) 2728282

Type:	30 ton travel hoist into locked marina basin
Suits:	larger craft
Availability:	all states of tide 0845 -1730 by prior arrangement
Restrictions:	dead slow in marina: no pwc; 6 mph speed limit in river
Facilities:	fuel, parking for car and trailer, toilets, showers and chandlery on site; locked marina entrance accessible at all times

Dues:	none
Charge:	approx. £50
Directions:	follow signs from A 19 trunk road/ Tyne Tunnel: site is 7 miles east of Newcastle
Waters accessed:	River Tyne and North Sea

North Shields (River Tyne) - Ferry Slipway
Tel: (0191) 2592499 (Mr Hardaker)

Type:	concrete slipway
Suits:	all craft
Availability:	approx. 3-4 hours either side HW (all states for small craft) by prior arrangement
Restrictions:	6 mph speed limit in river
Facilities:	fuel nearby, parking for car and trailer, toilets, water, chandlery, boat park and moorings on site
Dues:	none
Charge:	approx. £1
Directions:	follow A1058 from Newcastle-upon-Tyne: site is adjacent to North Shields ferry landing
Waters accessed:	River Tyne and North Sea

Cullercoats - Harbour Slip
Tel: (0191) 2621053 (Harbour Master)

Type:	concrete slipway into harbour
Suits:	dinghies and small powered craft
Availability:	approx. 2-3 hours either side HW
Restrictions:	5 knot speed limit inshore: water-skiing prohibited in harbour; site is staffed Whitsun to end Sept and may be congested
Facilities:	fuel from garage, parking for car in public car park nearby (c) and for trailer on site, toilets
Dues:	none
Charge:	craft under 10hp - £5 (£24 p.a.), craft over 10hp - £6 (£36 p.a.)
Directions:	follow A1058 east from Newcastle-upon-Tyne to Cullercoats
Waters accessed:	North Sea

Seaton Sluice Harbour
Tel: (01670) 542346 (Blyth Valley Council)

Type:	two steep concrete slipways
Suits:	all craft up to approx. 30'/9m LOA
Availability:	approx. 2 hours either side HW by prior arrangement
Restrictions:	5 mph speed limit in harbour and fairway: harbour has narrow entrance; permission to launch must be obtained by telephone - harbour is not manned; access to site is via narrow road and locked barrier
Facilities:	fuel from garage nearby, parking for car and trailer on site, toilets nearby, boat storage area, moorings available

Dues:	approx. £7
Charge:	no additional charge
Directions:	site is off A 193 between Blyth and Whitley Bay
Waters accessed:	North Sea

Newbiggin-by-the-Sea - Church Point Access, Pant Road
Tel: (01670) 819802 (Wansbeck D.C.)

Type:	concrete slipway onto hard wet sand
Suits:	all craft
Availability:	all states of tide
Restrictions:	10 mph speed limit within 50m of shoreline: occasional build-up of wind-blown sand normally removed within 48 hours; trailers and vehicles must not be left on beach
Facilities:	fuel from local garage, parking for car and trailer on site, toilets nearby, mobile countryside service on site at weekends
Dues:	none
Charge:	none
Directions:	follow A197 to coast from A1 at Morpeth: access is via Pant Road, next to Church Point car park
Waters accessed:	North Sea

Amble - The Braid
Tel: (01665) 710306 (Harbour Master)

Type:	concrete slipway
Suits:	small to medium-sized craft
Availability:	approx. 2-3 hours either side HW
Restrictions:	4 mph speed limit in harbour; water-skiing by arrangement with Harbour Master
Facilities:	fuel, parking for car and trailer and toilets on site: chandlery and yard facilities available at boatyard nearby
Dues:	approx. £5.25 daily or £40.50 for annual permit
Charge:	none
Directions:	follow A1068 north towards Alnwick, turning off between Amble and Warkworth: site is adjacent to Marina
Waters accessed:	North Sea

Beadnell
Tel: (01665) 721259 (Berwick-upon-Tweed B.C.)

Type:	shallow concrete ramp onto firm sandy beach
Suits:	craft which can be manhandled: tractor assistance available for larger craft (c)
Availability:	approx. 2-3 hours either side HW
Restrictions:	8 knot speed limit: water-skiing allowed offshore; launching is controlled by car park attendant 0830-1800
Facilities:	fuel from local garage, parking for car and trailer (c), toilets and showers (c) in car park

Dues:	none
Charge:	approx. £4.50 per day, £41.50 p.a.
Directions:	follow B1340 north from Alnwick: site is adjacent to car park
Waters accessed:	North Sea

Seahouses (North Sunderland) - Harbour Slipway
Tel: (01665) 720033 (Harbour Master)

Type:	concrete slipway onto sand
Suits:	small craft up to 25'/7.6m LOA
Availability:	all states of tide except 1 hour either side LWS 0845-1830
Restrictions:	3 knot speed limit in harbour: pwc not encouraged; craft must keep clear of ferries to Farne Islands; locked barrier to site and narrow access road down hill to harbour; slip is used to lauch Lifeboat and must be kept clear at all times; site can be dangerous in adverse weather conditions when barrier is closed and danger flags flying
Facilities:	fuel from local garage, parking for car in parking area (c) and for trailer on beach, toilets nearby, moorings in outer harbour and boat park with nightwatchman at weekends in summer
Dues:	none
Charge:	approx. £6 for boat and up to 2 persons, additional persons charged at £1 per head
Directions:	follow B1340 north from Alnwick
Waters accessed:	North Sea

Berwick-upon-Tweed - West End Road, Tweedmouth
Tel: (01289) 307404 (Harbour Master)

Type:	concrete slipway onto shingle
Suits:	small craft
Availability:	approx. 2½ hours either side HW
Restrictions:	6 knot speed limit; water-skiing and pwc prohibited
Facilities:	fuel from local garage, parking for car and trailer on roadside only, toilets
Dues:	none
Charge:	none
Directions:	turn off A1: site is adjacent old bridge on south side of River Tweed
Waters accessed:	North Sea

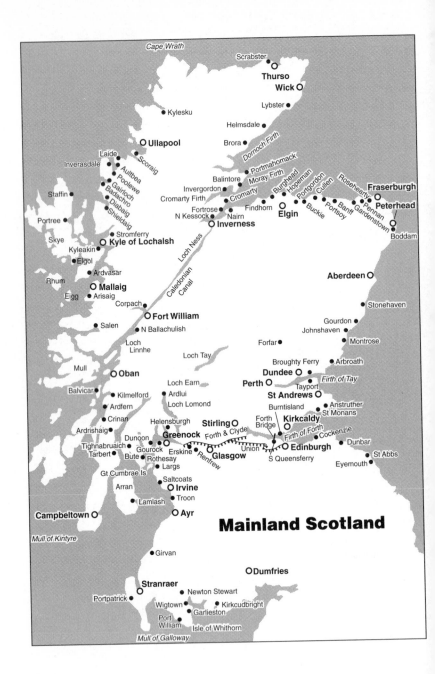

Mainland Scotland

Cape Wrath

Scrabster
Thurso O
Wick O
Lybster ●
Helmsdale ●
Kylesku ●
Brora ●
O Ullapool
Portmahomack
Laide ● Scoraig
Inverasdale ● Balintore
Aultbea Moray Firth Burghead
Poolewe Invergordon Hopeman Portgordon
Gairloch ● Cromarty Firth Cromarty Cullen Rosehearty
Staffin ● Badachro Fortrose ● Findhorn Portsoy Banff Pennan O Fraserburgh
Diabaig N Kessock ● Nairn Buckie Gardenstown Peterhead
Portree ● Shieldaig O Inverness Elgin
Boddam
Skye Stromferry
O Kyle of Lochalsh
Kyleakin ●
● Elgol Aberdeen O
Ardvasar
Rhum Caledonian Canal Stonehaven
O Mallaig Loch Ness
Eigg ● Arisaig Gourdon ●
Corpach Johnshaven ●
O Fort William Montrose
Salen ● N Ballachulish Forfar ● Arbroath
Loch Broughty Ferry ● St Monans
Linnhe Dundee O Anstruther
Loch Tay Perth O
Mull Tayport Firth of Tay
O Oban Loch Earn St Andrews O
Balvicar ● Ardlui Burntisland
Kilmelford ● Loch Lomond
Ardfern ● Forth Kirkcaldy
Crinan ● Helensburgh ● Stirling O Bridge Cockenzie
Ardrishaig ● Dunoon ● Greenock Forth & Clyde St Abbs
Tighnabruaich ● Gourock ● Erskine Union Edinburgh O Dunbar
Tarbert ● Bute ● Rothesay Renfrew Glasgow S Queensferry Eyemouth ●
Gt Cumbrae Is Largs Firth of Forth
Arran Saltcoats
O Irvine
Lamlash ● Troon
O Ayr
Campbeltown O
Mull of Kintyre
Girvan ●
O Dumfries
Stranraer O
Portpatrick ● Newton Stewart
Wigtown ● Kirkcudbright
Port Garlieston ●
William Isle of Whithorn
Mull of Galloway

Eyemouth - Harbour Slipway

Tel: (01890) 750223 or 750248 (home)

Type:	steep concrete slipway
Suits:	all craft up to approx. 20'/6.1m LOA
Availability:	approx. 4 hours either side HW
Restrictions:	5 mph speed limit in harbour: water-skiing permitted offshore; notify Harbour Master before use
Facilities:	fuel nearby, parking for car and trailer and chandlery on site, toilets, diving supplies and outboard repairs available nearby
Dues:	approx. £2.35
Charge:	no separate fee
Directions:	follow A1 north from Berwick-upon-Tweed to Ayton, turning onto A1107 for 2 miles to Eyemouth
Waters accessed:	North Sea

St Abbs - Harbour Slipway

Tel: (018907) 71708 (Harbour Master)

Type:	concrete slipway onto hard gravel
Suits:	all craft
Availability:	all states of tide for most boats
Restrictions:	speed limit in harbour: water-skiing permitted offshore; no launching in onshore winds as site is very exposed
Facilities:	fuel from Coldingham (1½ miles), parking for car and trailer (c), toilets, limited chandlery in Eyemouth; popular area for divers
Dues:	approx. £10
Charge:	none
Directions:	follow A1 north from Berwick-upon-Tweed turning onto A1107 to Eyemouth, then B6438 at Coldingham: final approach to harbour is steep and narrow
Waters accessed:	North Sea

Dunbar - Harbour Slipway, Victoria Place

Tel: (01368) 863206 (Harbour Master)

Type:	slipway of stone pitching onto level rock and sand
Suits:	all craft up to 30'/9m LOA
Availability:	approx. 2 hours either side HW
Restrictions:	3 mph in harbour: site is rocky and exposed
Facilities:	fuel nearby, parking for car and trailer on site, toilets, chandlery and diving supplies nearby
Dues:	approx. £5.50
Charge:	approx. £5.50
Directions:	turn off A1 onto A1087 to Dunbar, turning right at 'T' junction at north end of High St
Waters accessed:	Firth of Forth and North Sea

North Berwick - West Bay Slip
Tel: (01620) 893333 (Harbour Master)

Type:	shallow concrete ramp onto rock and sand beach
Suits:	all craft
Availability:	all states of tide across sand
Restrictions:	5 mph speed limit within Bay area and Fairway
Facilities:	fuel nearby, parking for car nearby and trailer on site (overnight on request), toilets, showers and changing facilities. diving supplies and outboard repairs all available on site
Dues:	none
Charge:	approx. £6.30
Directions:	follow A 198 east from Edinburgh and signs to harbour in town
Waters accessed:	Firth of Forth and North Sea

Cockenzie - West Harbour
Tel: (01875) 812150

Type:	concrete ramp
Suits:	all craft
Availability:	approx. 3 hours either side HW by prior arrangement
Restrictions:	none
Facilities:	fuel nearby, parking for car and trailer nearby, boat repairs on site
Dues:	approx. £5
Charge:	none
Directions:	follow A1 east from Edinburgh for 10 miles then signs from A198
Waters accessed:	Firth of Forth and North Sea

Granton - Harbour Slipway
Tel: (0131) 555 8750 (Forth Ports Plc)

Type:	cobbled slipway
Suits:	small craft which can be manhandled
Availability:	approx. 1 hour either side HW
Restrictions:	a permit must be obtained in advance from Forth Ports Plc
Facilities:	fuel nearby, parking for car and trailer by arrangement, chandlery and yacht club nearby: visiting yachts can be craned into the harbour by arrangement with the Royal Forth Yacht Club Tel: (0131) 552 8560
Dues:	yes
Charge:	approx. £13.50 per ft up to 18'/5.5m LOA (min charge £40)
Directions:	leave M8 at junction 2 taking A8 to Edinburgh city centre then follow signs to Granton: site is on east side of Middle Pier
Waters accessed:	Firth of Forth and North Sea

Cramond (Firth of Forth) - Riverside Walk Slipway
Tel: (0131) 336 1356 (Cramond Boat Club)

Type:	concrete slipway
Suits:	craft up to 25'/7.6m LOA
Availability:	approx. 2 hours either side HW
Restrictions:	none
Facilities:	parking for car and trailer nearby (c), toilets
Dues:	not known
Charge:	yes
Directions:	leave M8 at junction 2, taking A8/A902 and minor roads to Cramond: site is at mouth of river on east bank adjacent Cramond Boat Club
Waters accessed:	Firth of Forth and North Sea

South Queensferry (Firth of Forth) - Port Edgar Marina
Tel: (0131) 331 3330 Fax: (0131) 331 4878

Type:	concrete slipway
Suits:	all craft up to 30'/9m LOA
Availability:	approx. 5 hours either side HW, 0830-2200 by prior arrangement
Restrictions:	3 knot speed limit in harbour: water-skiing permitted in designated area downstream
Facilities:	diesel on site, petrol (1 mile), parking for car and trailer, toilets, chandlery and other marina facilities all on site
Dues:	none
Charge:	approx. £1.70 up to 16'/4.9m LOA and £4.50 over 16'/4.9m LOA
Directions:	leave M8 at junction 1 taking A8000 and minor roads: site is just west of Forth Bridge and access is via Shore Road
Waters accessed:	Firth of Forth and North Sea

North Queensferry (Firth of Forth) - Town Pier
Tel: (01592) 413518 (Fife Council)

Type:	cobbled slipway
Suits:	all craft up to 25'/7.6m LOA
Availability:	approx. 3-4 hours either side HW
Restrictions:	water-skiing permitted in designated area downstream
Facilities:	no parking
Dues:	approx. £4.20
Charge:	approx. £8.40
Directions:	follow signs to North Queensferry after crossing Forth Bridge: site is at far end of Main St between road and rail bridges
Waters accessed:	Firth of Forth and North Sea

North Queensferry (Firth of Forth) - Railway Pier

Tel: (01592) 413518 (Fife Council)

Type:	shallow concrete ramp
Suits:	all craft except windsurfers
Availability:	approx. 3-4 hours either side HW
Restrictions:	low speed in harbour: water-skiing permitted in designated area downstream
Facilities:	fuel nearby, parking for car and trailer on site, toilets and chandlery nearby; Boat Club on site Tel: (01383) 415678
Dues:	approx. £4.20
Charge:	approx. £8.40
Directions:	follow signs to North Queensferry after crossing Forth Bridge: site is off to the right of Main St under the road bridge
Waters accessed:	Firth of Forth and North Sea

Aberdour (Firth of Forth) - Shore Road Slipway

Type:	concrete slipway onto beach
Suits:	all craft up to 20'/6.1m LOA
Availability:	approx. 2 hours either side HW
Restrictions:	narrow access to site
Facilities:	fuel nearby, limited parking for car and trailer, toilets nearby
Dues:	none
Charge:	none
Directions:	follow A921 east from the north side of the Forth Bridge: site is at corner of Shore Rd, 100m from harbour
Waters accessed:	Firth of Forth and North Sea

Burntisland (Firth of Forth) - Burntisland Beach

Type:	concrete slipway onto beach
Suits:	small craft
Availability:	all states of tide
Restrictions:	none known
Facilities:	fuel nearby, parking for car and trailer, toilets, chandlery nearby
Dues:	none
Charge:	none
Directions:	follow A921 east from north side of Forth Bridge
Waters accessed:	Firth of Forth and North Sea

St Monan's (Firth of Forth) - Harbour Slipway

Tel: (01333) 310836 (0900-1700 mon to fri - Anstruther Harbour Master)

Type:	steep concrete ramp
Suits:	all craft except pwc and windsurfers
Availability:	approx. 2 hours either side HW
Restrictions:	low speed in harbour: access road is narrow
Facilities:	fuel from garage in Pittenweem, parking for car and trailer on site, boat repairs, toilets and chandlery nearby

Dues:	approx £8.40 (+ £4.20 per night)
Charge:	approx £8.40
Directions:	follow A917/B9131 south of St Andrews to Anstruther, then right onto A917, turning left to harbour between Elie and Pittenweem
Waters accessed:	Firth of Forth and North Sea

Anstruther (Firth of Forth) - Harbour Slipway

Tel: (01333) 310836 (0900-1700 mon to fri - Harbour Master)

Type:	concrete slipway (1:10)
Suits:	all craft up to 30'/9m LOA except pwc and windsurfers
Availability:	approx. 3 hours either side HW
Restrictions:	low speed in harbour
Facilities:	fuel nearby, parking for car and trailer (c), toilets and showers on site; chandlery from Pittenweem
Dues:	approx £8.40 (+ £4.20 per night)
Charge:	approx £8.40
Directions:	follow A917/B9131 south of St Andrews
Waters accessed:	Firth of Forth and North Sea

Cellardyke (Firth of Forth) - Harbour Slipway

Tel: (01333) 310836 (0900-1700 mon to fri - Harbour Master)

Type:	shallow cobbled ramp
Suits:	small sailing and powered craft except pwc
Availability:	approx. 3 hours either side HW, May to Sept only
Restrictions:	low speed in harbour: narrow entrance to harbour
Facilities:	petrol nearby, limited parking for car and trailer on site, toilets chandlery and diving supplies nearby
Dues:	approx £8.40 (+ £4.20 per night)
Charge:	approx £8.40
Directions:	turn off A917 coast road 1 mile east of Anstruther; access roads from Kilrenny are narrow and steep
Waters accessed:	Firth of Forth and North Sea

Crail (Firth of Forth) - Harbour Slipway, Shoregate

Tel: (01333) 450820 (part-time Harbour Master)

Type:	concrete ramp and cobbled slipway
Suits:	all craft except pwc
Availability:	approx. 3 hours either side HW
Restrictions:	2 mph speed limit when entering or leaving harbour: no pwc or windsurfers
Facilities:	fuel nearby, parking for car nearby and trailer on site, toilets, chandlery from Pittenweem (6 miles), outboard repairs in Methil (20 miles)
Dues:	approx £8.40
Charge:	none
Directions:	follow A917 south from St Andrews for 9 miles into centre of Crail: harbour is at bottom of Shoregate (narrow cul de sac)
Waters accessed:	Firth of Forth and North Sea

St Andrews - Harbour Slipway
Tel: (01334) 477107 (Harbour Trust)

Type:	shallow concrete and stone slipway
Suits:	small craft except pwc and windsurfers
Availability:	approx. 2 hours either side HW with Hb Mr's permission
Restrictions:	slow speed in harbour: narrow access
Facilities:	fuel in town, parking for car and trailer and toilets on site
Dues:	yes
Charge:	yes
Directions:	leave M90 at junction 8 taking the A917 east: follow signs through town to harbour: site is in corner of Outer Harbour
Waters accessed:	North Sea

Tayport (River Tay) - Harbour Slipway
Tel: (01382) 552249 (Tayport Harbour Trust)

Type:	slipway of concrete and cobbles
Suits:	all craft
Availability:	approx. 4 hours either side HW
Restrictions:	5 mph speed limit, advise Harbour Trust before launching
Facilities:	no diesel, petrol nearby, parking for car and trailer, toilets
Dues:	none
Charge:	approx. £4, £10 (week) or £25 (p.a.)
Directions:	leave M90 at junction 8 taking A91 east, then A914 following signs to Tay Bridge: turn right onto B946 before reaching bridge
Waters accessed:	River Tay, Firth of Tay and North Sea

Perth (River Tay) - Perth Water Ski Club, Shore Road
Tel: (01738) 630598 (Clubhouse)

Type:	medium concrete ramp into fresh water
Suits:	ski-boats and ribs: no pwc
Availability:	approx. 2 hours either side HW by prior arrangement
Restrictions:	site available to members only: locked barrier; insurance certificate required
Facilities:	fuel from garage nearby, parking for car and trailer, toilets, showers and changing rooms in clubhouse
Dues:	none
Charge:	yes
Directions:	leave M90 at junction 10 and follow signs to town centre: site is in Shore Road downstream of Queens Bridge and railway bridge
Waters accessed:	River Tay, Firth of Tay and North Sea

Kenmore - Loch Tay Boating Centre, Pier Road

Tel: (01887) 830291

Type:	shallow concrete slipway into non-tidal loch
Suits:	all craft except pwc
Availability:	0900 - 1900 Apr 1st to Oct 31st
Restrictions:	5 mph in harbour: pwc prohibited on Loch Tay; locked barrier outside hours
Facilities:	fuel nearby (6 miles), parking for car and trailer, toilets and outboard repairs all on site; tractor launch/ recovery available if required (c)
Dues:	approx. £6.50 per day
Charge:	no additional fee charged
Directions:	follow A9 north from Perth, turning left onto A827 to Aberfeldy and Kenmore and turning off in village: site is 100m from main road
Waters accessed:	Loch Tay

Tayside - Clatto Country Park

Tel: (01382) 436505 (Leisure & Parks Dept. Dundee City Council))

Type:	launching over foreshore into reservoir
Suits:	sailing dinghies and windsurfers: no powered craft
Availability:	1000-2000 mon & tues, 1000-1600 wed to sun
Restrictions:	powered craft prohibited
Facilities:	parking for car and trailer and toilets on site
Dues:	none
Charge:	approx. £3
Directions:	from Dundee take A923, crossing A972: at next round-about turn right, then next left and follow signs from Dalmahoy Drive
Waters accessed:	reservoir

Tayside - Monikie Country Park

Tel: (01382) 370202

Type:	launching into reservoir
Suits:	dinghies and small craft: no powered craft
Availability:	1000-2000 May - Aug, 1000 -1600 Sept and until 1 hour before dusk rest of year with day permit from Countryside Ranger
Restrictions:	powered craft prohibited
Facilities:	none known
Dues:	none
Charge:	approx. £3.50
Directions:	from Dundee take A92 east: turn left onto B962 and follow signs
Waters accessed:	lake/reservoir

Broughty Ferry - Harbour Slipway

Type:	concrete slipway
Suits:	dinghies
Availability:	approx. 4-5 hours either side HW
Restrictions:	5 knot speed limit inshore with access lane
Facilities:	not known
Dues:	none
Charge:	none
Directions:	follow A390 east from Dundee town centre for 3 miles
Waters accessed:	Firth of Tay and North Sea

Johnshaven - Harbour Slipway

Tel: (01561) 362262 (Harbour Master)

Type:	shallow concrete ramp into outer basin
Suits:	all shallow-draught craft
Availability:	approx. 3 hours either side HW by arrangement with Hbr Mr
Restrictions:	3 knot speed limit: water-skiing allowed outside harbour; narrow entrance through rocky foreshore can be difficult in winds between NE and SE
Facilities:	fuel nearby, parking for car and trailer, toilets and outboard repairs
Dues:	approx. £6
Charge:	no additional fee
Directions:	follow A92 north from Montrose
Waters accessed:	North Sea

Gourdon - Gourdon Harbour, Gourdon by Montrose

Tel: (01569) 762741 (Harbour Master)

Type:	two steep concrete slipways onto soft mud
Suits:	all craft up to approx. 18'/5.5m LOA except windsurfers and ski-boats
Availability:	approx. 3 hours either side of HW
Restrictions:	3 knot speed limit in harbour area: windsurfing and water-skiing prohibited; rocky harbour entrance - consult Hbr Mr before sailing; harbour should not be used in onshore winds, especially from SE
Facilities:	petrol nearby, diesel on fri a.m. from tanker, parking for car and trailer, small boat and diesel engine repairs all on site
Dues:	approx. £10
Charge:	no additional charge
Directions:	follow A 92 north from Montrose for 10 miles: road to harbour has steep hill and sharp bend at bottom of hill
Waters accessed:	North Sea

Stonehaven - Harbour Slipway

Tel: (01569) 762741 (Harbour Master)

Type:	concrete slipway onto hard sand in Inner Basin
Suits:	all craft up to approx. 18'/5.5m LOA except wind-surfers and ski-boats
Availability:	approx. 3 hours either side of HW
Restrictions:	3 knot speed limit in harbour: windsurfing and water-skiing prohibited; can be congested in summer; har-bour should not be used in winds from NE or E
Facilities:	petrol nearby, diesel on fri a.m. from tanker, parking for car and trailer and toilets and showers on site, pub nearby
Dues:	approx. £10
Charge:	no additional charge
Directions:	follow A90 south from Aberdeen for 15 miles and signs to harbour
Waters accessed:	North Sea

Boddam - Harbour Slipway

Tel: (01779) 478001

Type:	concrete slipway
Suits:	all craft
Availability:	all states of tide
Restrictions:	not known
Facilities:	petrol, parking for car only, toilets
Dues:	not known
Charge:	approx. £3
Directions:	turn off A952 south of Peterhead
Waters accessed:	North Sea

Peterhead - The Lido

Type:	concrete ramp onto firm sand
Suits:	sailing and small powered craft: no pwc, windsurfers or ski-boats
Availability:	all states of tide
Restrictions:	4 knot speed limit in marina: no pwc, windsurfing or water-skiing; access road is steep and fairly narrow
Facilities:	fuel nearby, parking for car and trailer and chandlery on site, toilets and outboard repairs nearby: berths in marina
Dues:	none
Charge:	none
Directions:	turn off A90 Aberdeen to Peterhead road to follow signs
Waters accessed:	Peterhead Bay Harbour and North Sea

Rosehearty - Harbour Slipway
Tel: (01346) 517599 (Harbour Master - part-time)

Type:	steep concrete slipway onto firm sand
Suits:	all craft up to 20'/6.1m LOA
Availability:	all states of tide except 1 hour either side of LWS
Restrictions:	3 knot speed limit in harbour: pwc prohibited but water-skiing permitted offshore; check with Harbour Master before launching; site is unsafe in onshore winds
Facilities:	fuel (4 miles), parking for car and trailer on site, toilets and chandlers nearby, pub, caravan site and golf course
Dues:	approx. £6
Charge:	none
Directions:	follow B9031 west from Fraserburgh for 4 miles
Waters accessed:	Moray Firth and North Sea

Pennan - Harbour Slipway
Tel: (01346) 561244 (Mrs Watt)

Type:	gentle concrete slipway onto sand and shingle
Suits:	dinghies and small powerboats
Availability:	approx. 2 hours either side of HW
Restrictions:	access to harbour is via steep road and site is very exposed especially in northerly winds
Facilities:	very limited parking for car and trailer, toilets
Dues:	approx. £4 for overnight mooring
Charge:	approx. £10
Directions:	follow B 9031 west from Fraserburgh for 4 miles
Waters accessed:	Moray Firth and North Sea

Gardenstown (Moray Firth) - Harbour Slipway
Tel: (01261) 851323 (Secretary, Harbour Trustees)

Type:	steep concrete slipway
Suits:	all craft up to 20'/6.1m LOA
Availability:	approx. 2 hours either side of HW
Restrictions:	5 mph speed limit in harbour and immediate surroundings: water-skiing allowed offshore; site unsuitable in northerly winds
Facilities:	petrol nearby, parking for car on site and trailer nearby, toilets on site, winch and pressure hose available by arrangement
Dues:	approx. £3.50
Charge:	no additional fee
Directions:	from Fraserburgh follow A98 and B9032/9031 west
Waters accessed:	Moray Firth and North Sea

Macduff (Moray Firth) - Harbour Slipway

Tel: (01261) 832236 (Harbour Master)

Type:	large shallow concrete ramp
Suits:	all shallow-draught craft
Availability:	approx. 3 hours either side of HW
Restrictions:	5 knot speed limit: water-skiing allowed outside harbour
Facilities:	fuel nearby, parking for car and trailer and toilets on site, chandlery, diving supplies and outboard repairs all nearby
Dues:	no additional fee
Charge:	approx. £8
Directions:	follow A950 west from Peterhead then A98: turn off main road with care
Waters accessed:	Moray Firth and North Sea

Banff (Moray Firth) - Harbour Slipway

Tel: (01261) 815544 (part-time Harbour Master - 24 hr answerphone)

Type:	shallow concrete slipway onto sand
Suits:	all craft up to approx. 30'/9m LOA except pwc
Availability:	approx. 3-4 hours either side HW: consult Harbour Master
Restrictions:	dead slow in harbour: no water-skiing, windsurfing or pwc within harbour limits; site is exposed in N to ENE winds
Facilities:	petrol nearby, diesel from Macduff, parking for car and trailer nearby, toilets on site, overnight berths (c), chandlery and outboard repairs nearby
Dues:	none
Charge:	approx. £10: 6 month ticket available (£45)
Directions:	follow A950 west from Peterhead then A98 or A947 from Aberdeen: turn off at bridge between Macduff and Banff: site is in Outer Basin at root of lighthouse pier
Waters accessed:	Moray Firth and North Sea

Portsoy (Moray Firth) - Harbour Slipway

Tel: (01261) 815544 (part-time Harbour Master - 24 hr answerphone)

Type:	steep concrete ramp
Suits:	all craft up to 30'/9m LOA except pwc
Availability:	approx. 3-4 hours either side HW: consult Harbour Master
Restrictions:	3 knot speed limit: no pwc, water-skiing or windsurfing within harbour limits
Facilities:	petrol in town, very limited parking for car and trailer, toilets
Dues:	none
Charge:	approx. £10: 6 month ticket available (£45)
Directions:	follow A950 west from Peterhead then A98 or A 947 from Aberdeen to Banff then A 98 Inverness road to Portsoy and signs to harbour: site is at east end of new harbour
Waters accessed:	Moray Firth and North Sea

Cullen (Moray Firth) - Harbour Slipway

Tel: (01261) 842477 (part-time Harbour Master)

Type:	steep concrete ramp onto soft sandy beach
Suits:	all craft up to 20'/6.1m LOA except pwc
Availability:	approx. 2 hours either side HW
Restrictions:	3 mph speed limit in harbour: site is very exposed in N to W winds; pwc prohibited
Facilities:	fuel nearby, parking for car and trailer and toilets on site
Dues:	approx. £6
Charge:	no separate fee
Directions:	follow A950 west from Peterhead then A98: site is at west end of harbour by West Pier
Waters accessed:	Moray Firth and North Sea

Portknockie (Moray Firth) - Inner Basin Slipway

Tel: (01542) 840833 (part-time Harbour Master)

Type:	steep tarmacadam ramp
Suits:	all craft
Availability:	approx. 4 hours either side HW
Restrictions:	3 knot speed limit in harbour: road to harbour is steep with tight u-bend near top of hill
Facilities:	fuel nearby, parking for car and trailer, toilets, water, electricity, shops, berths (c) all on site; other facilties nearby
Dues:	none
Charge:	approx. £7 (£28 per season)
Directions:	follow A96 east from Elgin turning off at Fochabers, then A98, turning left onto A942 and following signs to Portknockie after about 8 miles: site is in Inner Basin beside Middle Pier
Waters accessed:	Moray Firth and North Sea

Findochty (Moray Firth) - Harbour Slipway

Tel: (01542) 831466 (part-time Harbour Master)

Type:	long concrete slipway
Suits:	all craft up to approx. 25'/7.6m LOA
Availability:	approx. 2 hours either side HW
Restrictions:	dead slow speed limit in harbour: site is exposed in N winds when a swell can develop
Facilities:	fuel, parking for car and trailer, toilets nearby
Dues:	none
Charge:	approx. £8
Directions:	turn off A96 east of Elgin onto A98, turning left onto A942 and following coastal road: site is in Inner Basin by West Pier
Waters accessed:	Moray Firth and North Sea

Buckie (Cluny) (Moray Firth) - Harbour Slipway

Tel: (01542) 831700 (Harbour Master)

Type:	concrete ramp into No 4 Basin
Suits:	all craft up to 23'/7m LOA
Availability:	approx. 2 hours either side HW by prior arrangement
Restrictions:	3 mph speed limit in harbour
Facilities:	fuel nearby, parking for car and trailer on site, toilets and chandlery nearby; crane and winch for hire
Dues:	none
Charge:	approx. £7 or £26 unlimited use 1st Apr-30th Sept
Directions:	follow A96 east of Elgin, taking A98 and turning left after 7 miles onto A942
Waters accessed:	Moray Firth and North Sea

Portgordon (Moray Firth) - Harbour Slipway

Tel: (01343) 823000 (Mr Mark Fogden)

Type:	concrete slipway
Suits:	all craft
Availability:	approx. 2-3 hours either side HW
Restrictions:	none known
Facilities:	fuel from local garage, parking for car and trailer adjacent
Dues:	none
Charge:	none
Directions:	turn off A96 east of Elgin, taking A98 and turning onto A990: site is on east side of harbour
Waters accessed:	Moray Firth and North Sea

Hopeman (Moray Firth) - Harbour Slipway

Tel: (01343) 835337 (Harbour Master)

Type:	steep concrete slipway
Suits:	all craft
Availability:	approx. 2 hours either side HW with prior permission
Restrictions:	3 knot speed limit in harbour
Facilities:	fuel from garage (1/2 mile), parking for car and trailer, toilets and chandlery all on site
Dues:	none
Charge:	approx. £7 + vat
Directions:	follow A96 east from Inverness, turning onto B9013 between Forres and Elgin then right onto B9012 for 2 miles: site is in Inner Basin near West Pier
Waters accessed:	Moray Firth and North Sea

Burghead - Harbour Slipway

Tel: (01343) 835337 (Harbour Master)

Type:	steep concrete slipway 10'/3m wide onto sandy beach
Suits:	all craft up to 30'/9m LOA
Availability:	approx. 3 hours either side HW

Restrictions:	3 knot speed limit in harbour: narrow access road; this is a commercial and not a recreational harbour
Facilities:	fuel (2 miles), parking for car and trailer and toilets on site, water, electricity, crane for hire, chandlery & outboard repairs (3 miles)
Dues:	none
Charge:	approx. £7 + vat
Directions:	follow A 96 east from Inverness, turning onto B9013 between Forres and Elgin: site is near North Pier
Waters accessed:	Moray Firth and North Sea

Findhorn (Moray Firth) - Findhorn Boatyard

Tel: (01309) 690099

Type:	concrete slipway
Suits:	all craft
Availability:	all states of tide
Restrictions:	none
Facilities:	fuel from Kinloss, parking for car and trailer (c), toilets nearby, chandlers, repairs and diving supplies: 12 ton boat hoist, winter storage and cafe all on site: Royal Findhorn Y.C. and 2 water-ski clubs nearby
Dues:	none
Charge:	approx. £6.50
Directions:	follow A96 east from Inverness, turning onto B9011 at Forres then left at Kinloss following road through village
Waters accessed:	Moray Firth and North Sea

Nairn (Moray Firth) - Harbour Slipway

Tel: (01667) 454330 (Harbour Master)

Type:	shallow ramp with 4'6"/1.4m drop at end
Suits:	ribs, dinghies and small trailer sailers: no pwc
Availability:	approx. 1 hour either side HW
Restrictions:	5 knot speed limit in harbour: no pwc
Facilities:	fuel nearby, parking for car and trailer on site, toilets nearby, windsurfing supplies
Dues:	none
Charge:	yes
Directions:	take A96 Inverness to Aberdeen road turning down Harbour Street to the harbour
Waters accessed:	Moray Firth and North Sea

Inverness (Caledonian Canal) - Tomnahurich Bridge

Tel: (01463) 233140 (Canal Office)

Type:	steep slipway into approx. 5'/1.5m water
Suits:	small craft only
Availability:	during working hours 0800-1730 daily
Restrictions:	6 mph speed limit on canal: contact Canal Office prior to arrival to discuss requirements
Facilities:	fuel nearby, parking for car and trailer by arrangement, toilets, chandlery and outboard repairs nearby

Dues:	obtain BW licence from office
Charge:	none
Directions:	follow A9 to Inverness, then turn onto A82 and turn right at Tomnahurich Bridge
Waters accessed:	Caledonian Canal and Loch Ness

Inverness (Caledonian Canal) - Caley Marina, Canal Road
Tel: (01463) 236539

Type:	fairly steep slipway into 6'/1.8m water
Suits:	craft up to 21'/6.4m LOA except pwc
Availability:	0900-1730 mon to sat by prior arrangement
Restrictions:	6 mph speed limit in canal
Facilities:	diesel, petrol nearby, parking for car and trailer (c), toilets, overnight moorings, chandlery, engine repairs and boatyard with crane by arrangement
Dues:	obtain BW licence from office
Charge:	approx. £5
Directions:	leave A9 following signs for the A862 across Inverness to Muirtown swing bridge: turn up canal road by the flight of locks
Waters accessed:	Caledonian Canal and Loch Ness

South Kessock (Beauly Firth) - Old Ferry Pier

Type:	concrete slipway
Suits:	all craft up to 20'/6.1m LOA
Availability:	approx. 3 hours either side HW
Restrictions:	slip must be kept clear at all times for lifeboat launching
Facilities:	fuel, parking for car and trailer
Dues:	none
Charge:	none
Directions:	turn off A82 in Inverness: site is on south shore of Beauly Firth upstream of bridge:
Waters accessed:	Beauly Firth, Moray Firth and North Sea

North Kessock (Beauly Firth) - Old Ferry Pier
Tel: (01349) 865260 (Roads & Transport Div. Ross & Cromarty Area)

Type:	two concrete slipways
Suits:	all craft up to 20'/6.1m LOA
Availability:	approx. 3 hours either side HW
Restrictions:	none known
Facilities:	fuel, parking for car and trailer, toilets, chandlers on site
Dues:	payable to Highland Council - contact number above
Charge:	none
Directions:	follow A9 north from Inverness: site is on north shore of Beauly Firth upstream of bridge: site is adjacent Inverness Boat Centre (Tel: (01463) 731383)
Waters accessed:	Beauly Firth, Moray Firth and North Sea

Fortrose Harbour (Moray Firth) - Chanonry Sailing Club Slipway

Tel: (01381) 620861 (Harbour Master): (01381) 621973 (Clubhouse)

Type:	two concrete ramps
Suits:	all craft up to 20'/6.1m LOA except pwc
Availability:	approx. 3 hours either side HW
Restrictions:	6 knot speed limit in harbour
Facilities:	very limited parking for car, toilets nearby, chandlery and other facilities in Inverness or Kessock
Dues:	approx. £3
Charge:	visiting members £10 inc. use of slipway
Directions:	follow A9 north from Inverness, over Kessock Bridge then A832 to Fortrose/Cromarty
Waters accessed:	Moray Firth and North Sea

Fortrose (Moray Firth) - Chanonry Point Slipway

Tel: (01349) 865260 (Roads & Transport Div. Ross & Cromarty Area)

Type:	masonry slip
Suits:	all craft up to 20'/6.1m LOA
Availability:	approx. 3 hours either side HW
Restrictions:	none known
Facilities:	car parking
Dues:	as per Highland Council schedule of rates and dues - contact number above
Charge:	no separate fee charged
Directions:	follow A9 north from Inverness, over Kessock Bridge then A832 to Fortrose and turning onto minor roads to Chanonry Point
Waters accessed:	Moray Firth and North Sea

Balblair (Cromarty Firth) - Jetty

Tel: (01349) 865260 (Roads & Transport Div. Ross & Cromarty Area)

Type:	masonry slip
Suits:	all craft
Availability:	approx. 4 hours either side HW
Restrictions:	none known
Facilities:	none
Dues:	as per Highland Council schedule of rates and dues - contact number above
Charge:	no separate fee charged
Directions:	follow A9 north from Inverness, over Kessock Bridge then A832 to Fortrose and turning onto B9160 north to south shore of Cromarty Firth
Waters accessed:	Cromarty Firth, Moray Firth and North Sea

Invergordon (Cromarty Firth) - Rosskeen Slipway

Tel: (01349) 852308 (Cromarty Firth Port Authority)

Type:	shallow concrete ramp
Suits:	all craft except pwc
Availability:	approx. 3 hours either side HW
Restrictions:	8 knot speed limit in Cromarty Firth: water-skiing permitted with prior permission of Hbr Mr
Facilities:	fuel (2 miles), parking for car and trailer on site, toilets and chandlery (2 miles); Invergordon Boating Club clubhouse and boat pound adjacent - members only
Dues:	as per Highland Council schedule of rates and dues - (Tel: (01349) 865260)
Charge:	no separate fee charged
Directions:	follow A9 north from Inverness and along north shore of Cromarty Firth, turning off onto B817: site is half way between Alness and Invergordon
Waters accessed:	Cromarty Firth, Moray Firth and North Sea

Balintore (Moray Firth) - Harbour Slipway

Tel: (01349) 865260 (Roads & Transport Div. Ross & Cromarty Area)

Type:	concrete slipway onto hard sand
Suits:	all craft
Availability:	all states of tide
Restrictions:	none known
Facilities:	parking for car and trailer, toilets, chandlers, pontoon berths (c)
Dues:	as per Highland Council schedule of rates and dues - (Tel: (01349) 865260)
Charge:	no separate fee charged
Directions:	follow A9 north from Inverness, turning off south of Tain onto B9165/6
Waters accessed:	Moray Firth and North Sea

Hilton (Moray Firth) - The Slipway

Tel: (01349) 865260 (Roads & Transport Div. Ross & Cromarty Area)

Type:	concrete slipway
Suits:	all craft
Availability:	approx. 3 hours either side HW
Restrictions:	none known
Facilities:	limited parking in street, chandlers in Balintore
Dues:	as per Highland Council schedule of rates and dues - contact number above
Charge:	no separate fee charged
Directions:	follow A9 north from Inverness, turning off south of Tain onto B9165/6: site is 1 mile east of Balintore
Waters accessed:	Moray Firth and North Sea

Portmahomack (Dornoch Firth) - Harbour Slipway
Tel: (01862) 871705 (Harbour Master)

Type:	stone slipway into small drying harbour
Suits:	all craft up to 20'/6.1m LOA
Availability:	approx. 3 hours either side HW
Restrictions:	5 mph speed limit in harbour: contact Hbr Mr for permission
Facilities:	none on site
Dues:	as per Highland Council schedule of rates and dues - (Tel: (01349) 865260)
Charge:	no separate fee charged
Directions:	turn off south of Tain onto B9165
Waters accessed:	Dornoch Firth, Moray Firth and North Sea

Brora (Moray Firth) - Harbour Slipway

Type:	concrete slipway with heavy-duty hand winch
Suits:	all craft
Availability:	approx. 2½ hours either side HW
Restrictions:	none known
Facilities:	diesel on site, petrol (¼ mile), parking for car and trailer (c), chandlers and boatyard adjacent to slipway
Dues:	not known
Charge:	yes
Directions:	follow A9 north from Inverness, then minor road south of bridge to river mouth
Waters accessed:	Moray Firth and North Sea

Helmsdale (Moray Firth) - Harbour Slipway
Tel: (01431) 821386 (Harbour Master)

Type:	concrete slipway
Suits:	craft up to approx. 18'/5.5m LOA
Availability:	approx. 3 hours either side HW by prior arrangement
Restrictions:	speed limit in harbour: water-skiing permitted offshore, contact Harbour Master
Facilities:	fuel, parking for car and trailer and toilets nearby
Dues:	yes
Charge:	yes
Directions:	follow A9 north, turning right north of Helmsdale river bridge into Dunrobin St: take next right down to Shore St, then left: site is at east end of harbour
Waters accessed:	Moray Firth and North Sea

Lybster (Moray Firth) - Harbour Slipway

Type:	wooden ramp
Suits:	all craft
Availability:	approx. 2 hours either side HW
Restrictions:	slow speed in harbour: site exposed in onshore winds

Facilities:	fuel nearby, parking for car and trailer
Dues:	none
Charge:	none
Directions:	follow A9 south from Wick, turning off to village and harbour
Waters accessed:	Moray Firth and North Sea

Thurso Bay (Pentland Firth) - Scrabster

Tel: (01847) 892779 (Scrabster Harbour Trust)

Type:	concrete slipway
Suits:	all craft up to 25'/7.6m LOA
Availability:	approx. 3 hours either side HW
Restrictions:	5 knot speed limit in harbour
Facilities:	diesel on site, petrol (1½ miles), parking for car and trailer (c), toilets, chandlery, diving supplies and outboard repairs all nearby
Dues:	none
Charge:	none
Directions:	follow A882 north west from Wick: site is on west side of Thurso Bay
Waters accessed:	Pentland Firth

Kylesku South - Ferry Slipway

Type:	concrete slipway
Suits:	all craft
Availability:	approx. 5 hours either side HW
Restrictions:	none
Facilities:	parking for car & trailer and toilets nearby
Dues:	yes
Charge:	yes
Directions:	from Ullapool follow A835, A837 and A894 north: site is at south side of old ferry crossing
Waters accessed:	Locha'Chairn Bhain, Loch Glendhu and Loch Glencoul

Old Dornie

Tel: (01349) 865260 (Roads & Transport Div. Ross & Cromarty Area)

Type:	concrete slip
Suits:	all craft up to 20'/6.1m LOA
Availability:	approx. 3 hours either side HW
Restrictions:	none known
Facilities:	parking for car and trailer
Dues:	as per Highland Council schedule of rates and dues - contact number above
Charge:	no separate fee charged
Directions:	turn off A835 north of Ullapool onto the Achiltibuie road and turn off right onto minor road
Waters accessed:	Inner Minch and Summer Isles

Ullapool (Loch Broom) - Harbour Slipway

Type:	gentle concrete slipway
Suits:	all craft up to 18'/5.5m LOA
Availability:	approx. 5 hours either side HW
Restrictions:	4 knot speed limit in harbour
Facilities:	limited parking; Loch Broom S.C. nearby
Dues:	none
Charge:	none
Directions:	from Inverness follow A9 and A835 north to Ullapool
Waters accessed:	Loch Broom and The Minch

Scoraig (Little Loch Broom)

Tel: (01349) 865260 (Roads & Transport Div. Ross & Cromarty Area)

Type:	masonry ramp
Suits:	all craft up to 18'/5.5m LOA
Availability:	approx. 3 hours either side HW
Restrictions:	none known
Facilities:	none
Dues:	as per Highland Council schedule of rates and dues - contact number above
Charge:	no separate fee charged
Directions:	by sea only from Badluarach
Waters accessed:	Little Loch Broom

Badluarach

Tel: (01349) 865260 (Roads & Transport Div. Ross & Cromarty Area)

Type:	masonry slip
Suits:	all craft up to 20'/6.1m LOA
Availability:	approx. 3 hours either side HW
Restrictions:	none known
Facilities:	none
Dues:	as per Highland Council schedule of rates and dues - contact number above
Charge:	no separate fee charged
Directions:	from Inverness follow A9 and A835 north then A832 west to south shore of Little Loch Broom
Waters accessed:	Gruinard Bay

Laide

Tel: (01349) 865260 (Roads & Transport Div. Ross & Cromarty Area)

Type:	stone and concrete slipway
Suits:	small craft
Availability:	approx. 3 hours either side HW
Restrictions:	none known
Facilities:	limited parking for car, leave trailer by arrangement
Dues:	as per Highland Council schedule of rates and dues - contact number above

Charge:	no separate fee charged
Directions:	from Inverness follow A9 and A835 north then A832 west to west shore of Gruinard Bay: site is 1/2 mile from Post Office
Waters accessed:	Gruinard Bay

Aultbea (Loch Ewe)

Tel: (01349) 865260 (Roads & Transport Div. Ross & Cromarty Area)

Type:	stone and concrete slipway
Suits:	small craft
Availability:	approx. 3 hours either side HW
Restrictions:	none known
Facilities:	fuel, limited parking for car, leave trailer by arrangement, toilets
Dues:	as per Highland Council schedule of rates and dues - contact number above
Charge:	no separate fee charged
Directions:	from Inverness follow A9 and A835 north then A832 west to east side of Loch Ewe: site is near Aultbea Hotel
Waters accessed:	Loch Ewe

Poolewe (Loch Ewe)

Type:	stone and concrete slipway
Suits:	small craft
Availability:	all states of tide except LWS
Restrictions:	none known
Facilities:	limited parking for car and trailer by arrangement
Dues:	none
Charge:	none
Directions:	from Inverness follow A9 and A835 north then A832 west to south side of Loch Ewe
Waters accessed:	Loch Ewe

Inverasdale (Loch Ewe)

Tel: (01349) 865260 (Roads & Transport Div. Ross & Cromarty Area)

Type:	masonry ramp
Suits:	small craft only
Availability:	3 hours either side HW
Restrictions:	difficult access road: a new pier and concrete slip are soon to be built together with access road and car park
Facilities:	none
Dues:	as per Highland Council schedule of rates and dues - contact number above
Charge:	no separate fee charged
Directions:	from Inverness follow A9 and A835 north then A832 west to Poolewe and B8057 north to west side of Loch Ewe
Waters accessed:	Loch Ewe

Strath, Gairloch (Loch Gairloch)

Tel: (01349) 865260 (Roads & Transport Div. Ross & Cromarty Area)

Type: stone and concrete slipway
Suits: small craft up to 18'/5.5m LOA
Availability: all states of tide except LWS
Restrictions: none known
Facilities: none
Dues: as per Highland Council schedule of rates and dues - contact number above
Charge: no separate fee charged
Directions: from Inverness follow A9 and A835 north then A832 west to Gairloch: turn onto B8021: site is on north shore of Loch Gairloch
Waters accessed: Loch Gairloch

Gairloch (Loch Gairloch) - Pier Road

Tel: (01445) 712140 (Pier Master)

Type: tarmac surface over rock
Suits: all craft up to 30'/9m LOA
Availability: approx. 3 hours either side HW or HW only for larger craft
Restrictions: no speed limit, water-skiing permitted provided fishing boats not obstructed: contact Hbr Mr for further information
Facilities: fuel at pier by arrangement, parking for car and trailer, toilets, chandlery, repairs and engineering: temporary membership of club adjacent to slipway allows use of facilities
Dues: as per Highland Council schedule of rates and dues - contact number above
Charge: no separate fee charged
Directions: from Inverness follow A9 and A835 north then A832 west to Gairloch: site is on east side of Loch Gairloch
Waters accessed: Loch Gairloch

Badachro (Loch Gairloch)

Tel: (01349) 865260 (Roads & Transport Div. Ross & Cromarty Area)

Type: stone and concrete slipway
Suits: all craft up to 20'/6.1m LOA
Availability: approx. 3 hours either side HW
Restrictions: none known
Facilities: parking for car, leave trailer by arrangement
Dues: as per Highland Council schedule of rates and dues - contact number above
Charge: no separate fee charged
Directions: from Inverness follow A9 and A835 north then A832 west and turn onto B8056 to south shore of Loch Gairloch
Waters accessed: Loch Gairloch

Inveralligin (Upper Loch Torridon)

Tel: (01349) 865260 (Roads & Transport Div. Ross & Cromarty Area)

Type:	masonry slip
Suits:	small craft
Availability:	approx. 3 hours either side HW
Restrictions:	none known
Facilities:	none
Dues:	as per Highland Council schedule of rates and dues - contact number above
Charge:	no separate fee charged
Directions:	take A896 fron Lochcarron, turning left at Torridon onto minor road
Waters accessed:	Upper Loch Torridon

Diabaig (Loch Torridon)

Tel: (01349) 865260 (Roads & Transport Div. Ross & Cromarty Area)

Type:	steep concrete ramp
Suits:	small powered and sailing craft up to 16'/4.9m LOA
Availability:	all states of tide
Restrictions:	remote site at end of narrow single-track road with very steep hills (1:3) and hairpin bends - need 4x4 vehicle for access
Facilities:	parking for car and trailer
Dues:	as per Highland Council schedule of rates and dues - contact number above
Charge:	no separate fee charged
Directions:	turn off A896 at head of loch onto single track road
Waters accessed:	Outer Loch Torridon and sea

Shieldaig (Loch Torridon)

Tel: (01349) 865260 (Roads & Transport Div. Ross & Cromarty Area)

Type:	concrete slip
Suits:	all craft up to 20'/6.1m LOA
Availability:	approx. 3 hours either side HW
Restrictions:	none known
Facilities:	none
Dues:	as per Highland Council schedule of rates and dues - contact number above
Charge:	no separate fee charged
Directions:	follow A896 to Shieldaig from Lochcarron
Waters accessed:	Loch Torridon

North Strome (Loch Carron)

Tel: (01599) 534167 (Harbour Master, Kyle)

Type:	concrete slipway
Suits:	all craft up to 20'/6.1m LOA
Availability:	all states of tide
Restrictions:	none known
Facilities:	parking for car and trailer

Dues:	as per Highland Council schedule of rates and dues
Charge:	approx. £5
Directions:	from Fort William take A82 north to Invergarry then A87 west and A890 north east, turning west onto A896 at Strathcarron and following minor road west of Lochcarron: site is at old ferry site on north shore of Loch Carron
Waters accessed:	Loch Carron and Inner Sound

Stromeferry (Loch Carron) - Old Ferry Stage

Tel: (01599) 534167 (Harbour Master, Kyle)

Type:	concrete slipway
Suits:	all craft up to 20'/6.1m LOA
Availability:	all states of tide
Restrictions:	none known
Facilities:	parking for car and trailer
Dues:	as per Highland Council schedule of rates and dues
Charge:	approx. £5
Directions:	from Fort William take A82 north to Invergarry then A87 west and A890 north: site is at old ferry site on south shore of Loch Carron
Waters accessed:	Loch Carron and Inner Sound

Dornie (Loch Long)

Tel: (01599) 534167 (Harbour Master, Kyle)

Type:	flagstone
Suits:	small craft
Availability:	approx. 2 hours either side HW
Restrictions:	light trailers only
Facilities:	none
Dues:	as per Highland Council schedule of rates and dues
Charge:	approx. £5
Directions:	situated adjacent to west end of Dornie Bridge on A87
Waters accessed:	Loch Long, Loch Duich, Loch Alsh and Inner Sound

Plockton (Loch Carron)

Tel: (01599) 534167 (Harbour Master, Kyle)

Type:	stone jetty with irregular surface
Suits:	small craft
Availability:	approx. 2 hours either side HW
Restrictions:	dog-leg in middle of slip
Facilities:	none
Dues:	as per Highland Council schedule of rates and dues
Charge:	approx. £5
Directions:	from Fort William take A82 north to Invergarry then A87 west and A890 north, then minor road west to Plockton: site is at entrance to Loch Carron
Waters accessed:	Loch Carron and Inner Sound

Kyle of Lochalsh (Loch Alsh) - Old Ferry Slipway
Tel: (01599) 534167 (Harbour Master, Kyle)

Type:	graduated concrete slipway
Suits:	all craft
Availability:	all states of tide
Restrictions:	contact Harbour Master (ferry office) for permission to launch
Facilities:	fuel nearby, parking for car and trailer, toilets
Dues:	as per Highland Council schedule of rates and dues
Charge:	approx. £5
Directions:	from Fort William take A82 north to Invergarry then A87 west
Waters accessed:	Loch Alsh and Inner Sound

Balmacara (Loch Alsh)
Tel: (01599) 534167 (Harbour Master, Kyle)

Type:	graduated slipway
Suits:	small craft only
Availability:	approx. 3 hours either side of HW
Restrictions:	none known
Facilities:	shop, pub, hotel and post office nearby
Dues:	as per Highland Council schedule of rates and dues
Charge:	approx. £5
Directions:	from Fort William take A82 north to Invergarry then A87 west
Waters accessed:	Loch Alsh and Inner Sound

Shiel Bridge (Loch Duich)
Tel: (01599) 534167 (Harbour Master, Kyle)

Type:	stone slipway
Suits:	small craft only
Availability:	approx. 2 hours either side HW
Restrictions:	none known
Facilities:	fuel, parking for car and trailer
Dues:	as per Highland Council schedule of rates and dues
Charge:	approx. £5
Directions:	from Fort William take A82 north to Invergarry then A87 west: site is at head of loch opposite Kintail Lodge Hotel
Waters accessed:	Loch Duich, Loch Alsh and Inner Sound

Glenelg (Sound of Sleat)
Tel: (01599) 534167 (Harbour Master, Kyle)

Type:	graduated slipway
Suits:	small craft
Availability:	at all states of tide
Restrictions:	keep clear of Kylerhea Ferry
Facilities:	none

Dues:	as per Highland Council schedule of rates and dues
Charge:	approx. £5
Directions:	from Fort William take A82 north to Invergarry then A87 west to Shiel Bridge at head of Loch Duich: site is at end of minor road to the west
Waters accessed:	Glenelg Bay and Sound of Sleat

Isle of Skye, Kyleakin - Old Ferry Slipway

Tel: (01599) 534167 (Harbour Master, Kyle)

Type:	concrete slipway
Suits:	all craft
Availability:	all states of tide
Restrictions:	ferry must not be obstructed, contact Harbour Master at Kyle of Lochalsh
Facilities:	fuel nearby, parking for car and trailer
Dues:	as per Highland Council schedule of rates and dues
Charge:	approx. £5
Directions:	follow A87 south from Portree: site is adjacent ferry slip
Waters accessed:	Loch Alsh and Inner Sound

Isle of Skye - Broadford

Tel: (01478) 612926 (Harbour Office, Portree)

Type:	concrete slipway
Suits:	all craft
Availability:	all states of tide
Restrictions:	none
Facilities:	fuel, parking for car and trailer, toilets & stores nearby
Dues:	as per Highland Council schedule of rates and dues
Charge:	approx. £5
Directions:	follow A87 eight miles west from Skye Bridge
Waters accessed:	Broadford Bay and Inner Sound

Isle of Skye - Sconser

Tel: (01478) 612926 (Harbour Office, Portree)

Type:	concrete ferry slipway
Suits:	all craft
Availability:	all states of tide
Restrictions:	ferry must not be obstructed: contact Harbour Master
Facilities:	limited parking for car and trailer, toilets
Dues:	as per Highland Council schedule of rates and dues
Charge:	yes
Directions:	follow A87 west from Skye Bridge for 24 miles
Waters accessed:	Loch Sligachan, Sound of Raasay

Isle of Skye, Portree - Harbour Slipway

Tel: ((01478) 612926 (Harbour Office)

Type:	stone and concrete slipway
Suits:	all craft
Availability:	approx. 4-5 hours either side HW
Restrictions:	contact Harbour Master

Facilities:	fuel, parking for car and trailer, toilets and stores
Dues:	as per Highland Council schedule of rates and dues
Charge:	yes
Directions:	follow A87 north from Skye Bridge for 35 miles
Waters accessed:	Loch Portree, Sound of Raasay

Isle of Skye, Portree - Scorrybreac Slipway
Tel: (01478) 612926 (Harbour Office, Portree)

Type:	narrow concrete slipway in harbour
Suits:	all craft up to 16'/5m LOA
Availability:	approx. 4-5 hours either side HW
Restrictions:	contact Harbour Master
Facilities:	fuel, parking for car and trailer, toilets and stores
Dues:	as per Highland Council schedule of rates and dues
Charge:	yes
Directions:	follow A87 north from Skye Bridge for 35 miles
Waters accessed:	Loch Portree, Sound of Raasay

Isle of Skye - Staffin
Tel: (01478) 612926 (Harbour Office, Portree)

Type:	stone and concrete slipway
Suits:	all craft up to 33'/10m LOA
Availability:	all states of tide
Restrictions:	none
Facilities:	fuel, parking for car and trailer, stores
Dues:	as per Highland Council schedule of rates and dues
Charge:	yes
Directions:	follow A87 to Portree, then A855 (narrow road) north for approx. 20 miles
Waters accessed:	Staffin Bay

Isle of Skye - Kilmoluaig
Tel: (01478) 612926 (Harbour Office, Portree)

Type:	concrete slipway, all above MHWN onto beach
Suits:	small craft only
Availability:	approx. 1 hour either side HW
Restrictions:	none
Facilities:	parking for car and trailer
Dues:	as per Highland Council schedule of rates and dues
Charge:	yes
Directions:	follow A87 to Portree, then A855 (narrow road) north for approx. 25 miles
Waters accessed:	Little Minch

Isle of Skye - Camus Mor
Tel: (01478) 612926 (Harbour Office, Portree)

Type:	concrete slipway
Suits:	all craft up to 24'/7.5m LOA
Availability:	approx. 5 hours either side of HW
Restrictions:	none

Facilities:	parking for car and trailer
Dues:	as per Highland Council schedule of rates and dues
Charge:	yes
Directions:	follow A87 north to Portree, then A856 to Uig and A855 north
Waters accessed:	Loch Snizort and Little Minch

Isle of Skye - Uig

Tel: (01478) 612926 (Harbour Office, Portree)

Type:	concrete slipway in harbour
Suits:	small craft
Availability:	approx. 4-5 hours either side HW
Restrictions:	contact Harbour Master
Facilities:	fuel, parking for car and trailer, toilet, stores
Dues:	contact Harbour Master
Charge:	yes
Directions:	follow A87 north to Portree, then A 856 to Uig
Waters accessed:	Uig Bay, Loch Snizort and Little Minch

Isle of Skye - Stein, Waternish

Tel: (01478) 612926 (Harbour Office, Portree)

Type:	narrow concrete slipway
Suits:	all craft up to approx. 25'/7.5m LOA
Availability:	approx. 4-5 hours either side HW
Restrictions:	access is via narrow roads
Facilities:	limited parking for car and trailer
Dues:	as per Highland Council schedule of rates and dues
Charge:	yes
Directions:	from Portree follow A87 north west then B886: site is on western side of Waternish Peninsula, 55 miles from Skye Bridge
Waters accessed:	Loch Bay

Isle of Skye - Colbost Pier

Tel: (01478) 612926 (Harbour Office, Portree)

Type:	concrete slipway
Suits:	all craft up to 25'/7.5m LOA
Availability:	approx. 5 hours either side HW
Restrictions:	access is restricted
Facilities:	none
Dues:	as per Highland Council schedule of rates and dues
Charge:	yes
Directions:	follow A87 from Skye bridge until Borve, then take A850 for Dunvegan and B884 to Glendale: follow signs to Colbost Jetty on west side of loch
Waters accessed:	Loch Dunvegan

Isle of Skye - Glendale, Pooltiel

Tel: (01478) 612926 (Harbour Office, Portree)

Type:	concrete slipway
Suits:	all craft up to approx. 25'/7.5m LOA
Availability:	approx. 4-5 hours either side HW
Restrictions:	very narrow access roads
Facilities:	limited parking for car and trailer
Dues:	as per Highland Council schedule of rates and dues
Charge:	yes
Directions:	follow A87 west from Skye Bridge. turning onto A863 after Sconser, then turn left onto B884 at Lonmore
Waters accessed:	Loch Pooltiel and Neist Point

Isle of Skye - Caroy

Tel: (01478) 612926 (Harbour Office, Portree)

Type:	concrete slipway
Suits:	all craft up to approx. 25'/7.5m LOA
Availability:	approx. 4-5 hours either side HW
Restrictions:	none
Facilities:	limited parking for car and trailer
Dues:	as per Highland Council schedule of rates and dues
Charge:	yes
Directions:	follow A87 west from Skye Bridge, turning onto A863 after Sconser
Waters accessed:	Loch Bracadale

Isle of Skye - Elgol

Tel: (01478) 612926 (Harbour Office, Portree)

Type:	concrete slipway
Suits:	all craft
Availability:	at all states of tide
Restrictions:	none
Facilities:	parking for car and trailer, toilets
Dues:	as per Highland Council schedule of rates and dues
Charge:	yes
Directions:	follow A87 west from bridge, turning south onto B8083 in Broadford
Waters accessed:	Loch Scavaig

Isle of Skye - Ardvasar Bay (Sleat Marine Services)

Tel: (01471) 844216 Fax: (01471) 844387

Type:	shingle foreshore becoming sand
Suits:	all craft up to 30'/9m LOA except pwc
Availability:	approx. 3 hours either side HW: check for availability
Restrictions:	speed limit: slip may be obstructed
Facilities:	diesel on site, petrol nearby, parking for car and trailer, toilets & showers, limited chandlery and outboard repairs all on site
Dues:	none
Charge:	none

Directions:	from Portree follow A850 south to Broadford then A851
	or by ferry from Mallaig: site is opposite village stores
Waters accessed:	Sound of Sleat

Isle of Skye - Armadale

Tel: (01478) 612075 (Caledonian MacBrayne)

Type:	concrete slipway
Suits:	small craft
Availability:	all states of tide
Restrictions:	keep clear of Mallaig Ferry
Facilities:	fuel,shops and pub
Dues:	as per Highland Council schedule of rates and dues
Charge:	approx. £5
Directions:	follow A87 west from Skye Bridge, turning south onto A851
Waters accessed:	Sound of Sleat

Isle of Skye - Kylerhea Pier

Tel: (01599) 534167 (Harbour Master, Kyle)

Type:	graduated concrete slipway
Suits:	all craft
Availability:	at all states of tide
Restrictions:	keep clear of Glenelg Ferry
Facilities:	none
Dues:	as per Highland Council schedule of rates and dues
Charge:	approx. £5
Directions:	follow A87 from Skye bridge for 4 miles & then turn left for Kylerhea
Waters accessed:	Glenelg Bay and Sound of Sleat

Mallaig (Sound of Sleat) - Harbour Slipway

Tel: (01687) 462154 (Harbour Master)

Type:	narrow and fairly steep concrete slipway
Suits:	sailing dinghies, trailer-sailers and canoes
Availability:	approx. 3 hours either side HW
Restrictions:	speed limit: no water-skiing; narrow access
Facilities:	fuel nearby, parking for car and trailer on site, toilets, chandlers and outboard repairs nearby
Dues:	none
Charge:	none
Directions:	follow A830 west from Fort William: site is located south east from harbour adjacent to car park
Waters accessed:	Sound of Sleat

Arisaig Harbour (Sound of Sleat) - Arisaig Maritime Ltd
Tel: (01687) 450224

Type:	concrete slipway with rails
Suits:	all craft up to 20'/6.1m LOA
Availability:	approx. 4 hours either side HW 0900-1800
Restrictions:	water-skiing allowed with permission
Facilities:	diesel on site, parking for car and trailer, crane and winch for hire, toilets nearby, limited chandlery, repairs, moorings, shop, hotel, restaurant and accommodation
Dues:	included in launching fee
Charge:	approx. £4 + vat
Directions:	follow A830 west from Fort William; road has 12 1/2'/3.8m height restriction
Waters accessed:	Loch nan Ceall

Glenuig, by Lochailort - Glenuig Slipway
Tel: (01397) 703701 (Highland Council)

Type:	medium concrete ramp
Suits:	all craft up to 25'/7.6m LOA
Availability:	approx. 4 hours either side HW
Restrictions:	none
Facilities:	parking for car and trailer
Dues:	none
Charge:	approx. £3.50
Directions:	follow A861 south of Lochailort for 8 miles to south shore of Sound of Arisaig
Waters accessed:	Sound of Arisaig and open sea

Salen, nr Acharacle (Loch Sunart) - Salen Jetty
Tel: (01967) 431333

Type:	shingle foreshore into creek
Suits:	all craft
Availability:	all states of tide by arrangement on arrival
Restrictions:	low speed inshore
Facilities:	diesel on site, petrol (7 miles), parking for car and trailer (c), water, moorings, shops in village
Dues:	none
Charge:	approx. £10
Directions:	from Fort William either follow A830 west taking A861 at Lochailort and B8007 in Salen or take A82 south, crossing Loch Linnhe on Corran Ferry and follow A861 via Strontian to Salen: site is on north shore of Loch Sunart on the Ardnamurchan Peninsula
Waters accessed:	Loch Sunart and open sea

Acharacle (Loch Sunart) - Resipole Caravan Park
Tel: (01967) 431235 (Reception)

Type:	shallow concrete ramp
Suits:	all craft up to 20'/6.1m LOA
Availability:	approx. 3 hours either side HW by prior arrangement
Restrictions:	overhead telephone cable beside main road
Facilities:	fuel (7 miles), parking for car and trailer and toilets on site, self-contained accommodation, caravan park, restaurant and bar on site
Dues:	none
Charge:	approx. £5
Directions:	from Fort William follow either A830 west taking A861 at Lochailort or A82 south, crossing Loch Linnhe on Corran Ferry and taking A861 via Strontian: site is 8 miles west of Strontian
Waters accessed:	Loch Sunart and open sea

Strontian (Loch Sunart) - Loch Sunart Jetty
Tel: (01397) 703701 (Highland Council)

Type:	medium concrete ramp
Suits:	small craft
Availability:	approx. 3 hours either side HW
Restrictions:	none
Facilities:	parking for car and trailer
Dues:	none
Charge:	approx. £3.50
Directions:	follow A861 south from Lochailort: site is at head of loch and 1 mile east of Strontian village
Waters accessed:	Loch Sunart

Fort William (Loch Linnhe) - Lochaber Yacht Club, Achintore Road
Tel: (01397) 702370/772361

Type:	concrete ramp
Suits:	sailing dinghies and small trailer-sailers up to 25'/7.6m LOA
Availability:	approx. 5 hours either side HW by prior arrangement
Restrictions:	keep clear of all Y.C. launching and recovery activities
Facilities:	fuel (1 mile), parking for car & trailer (1/2 mile), toilets in clubhouse
Dues:	none
Charge:	donations welcome
Directions:	follow A82 south from Fort William town centre (1/2 mile): site is at junction with Ashburn Lane and access is steep
Waters accessed:	Loch Linnhe and Firth of Lorn

South Laggan (Loch Oich) - Monster Activities, Great Glen Water Park
Tel: (01809) 501340

Type:	steep concrete slipway into approx. 4'/1.2m water
Suits:	all craft up to 20'/6.1m LOA
Availability:	0900 - 2100 daily by prior arrangement
Restrictions:	6 mph speed limit in Caledonian Canal: none on Loch Oich
Facilities:	fuel nearby, parking for car and trailer (c), water, toilets, overnight moorings, boatyard, restaurant, self-catering accommodation and shop; full watersports centre and white-water rafting
Dues:	none for Loch Oich but obtain BW licence from Canal Office at Seaport Marina, Muirtown (Tel: (01463) 233140) for Caledonian Canal
Charge:	approx. £10
Directions:	from Fort William follow A82 north for 22 miles , turning right just before South Laggan swing bridge: site is at south west end of Loch Oich
Waters accessed:	Loch Oich and Caledonian Canal

North Ballachulish (Loch Leven) - Old Ferry slipway

Type:	concrete slipway
Suits:	all craft up to 20'/6.1m LOA
Availability:	approx. 5 hours either side HW
Restrictions:	strong current
Facilities:	fuel in village, very limited parking for car and trailer, hotels nearby
Dues:	none
Charge:	none
Directions:	follow A82 south from Fort William, turning left onto B863 before bridge then right into Old Ferry Rd and go to end, close to bridge
Waters accessed:	Loch Leven and Loch Linnhe

South Ballachulish (Loch Leven) - Laroch

Type:	concrete slipway
Suits:	all craft up to 25'/7.6m LOA
Availability:	approx. 5 hours either side HW
Restrictions:	strong current
Facilities:	fuel in village, limited parking for car and trailer, hotels nearby
Dues:	none
Charge:	none
Directions:	follow A82 south from Fort William, turn onto A828: site is underneath road bridge opposite Ballachulish Hotel
Waters accessed:	Loch Leven and Loch Linnhe

Kentallen (Loch Linnhe) - Holly Tree Hotel

Tel: (01631) 740292

Type:	concrete slipway
Suits:	all craft
Availability:	approx. 4 hours either side of HW
Restrictions:	use by prior arrangement with hotel proprietor
Facilities:	parking for car, leave trailer by arrangement with hotel, accommodation and restaurant
Dues:	none known
Charge:	none known
Directions:	follow A82 and A828 south from Fort William: site is 3 miles south of Ballachulish Bridge on east shore of Loch Linnhe near pier
Waters accessed:	Loch Linnhe

Oban, Barcaldine - Creran Moorings

Tel: (01631) 720265

Type:	shallow concrete ramp
Suits:	all craft up to 25'/7.6m LOA except pwc and wind-surfers
Availability:	all states of tide except for 1 hour either side LWS
Restrictions:	none
Facilities:	fuel (6 miles), parking for car and trailer (c), toilets and showers, moorings, camping, chalets/caravans to let
Dues:	none
Charge:	approx. £6
Directions:	from Oban follow A828 north: site is 1 mile north of Sea Life Centre
Waters accessed:	Loch Creran, Loch Linnhe and Scottish West Coast

Oban, Dunbeg - Dunstaffnage Marina

Tel: (01631) 566555

Type:	shallow block ramp
Suits:	all craft up to 30'/9m LOA except pwc
Availability:	approx. 2 hours either side HW by prior arrangement
Restrictions:	4 knot speed limit: water-skiing and pwc prohibited
Facilities:	diesel on site, petrol nearby, parking for car and trailer, toilets & showers, moorings, 18 ton travel lift, restaurant, shop and chandlery
Dues:	none known
Charge:	yes
Directions:	from Oban take A85 north for 3 miles
Waters accessed:	Firth of Lorn, Sound of Mull and Scottish West Coast

Oban, Ganavan Sands - Ganavan Sands Caravan Park

Tel: (01631) 562179

Type:	wide (40'/12.2m) concrete slipway
Suits:	small shallow-draught sailing and powered craft
Availability:	approx. 3 hours either side HW; report to site shop

Restrictions: 10 mph speed limit, water-skiing and pwc permitted offshore: locked barrier 2300-0600; no dogs allowed on site

Facilities: fuel (2 miles), parking for car and trailer (c), toilets, touring caravan site and small shop on site: chandlery, diving supplies and outboard repairs in Oban (2 miles)

Dues: none

Charge: approx. £3.50

Directions: entering Oban on the A82, go down hill and turn right at the second small roundabout; follow this road, keeping the sea on your left, for 2 miles

Waters accessed: Firth of Lorn, Loch Creran and Scottish West Coast

Oban - Railway Pier Slipway

Tel: (01631) 570802 (Pier Master)

Type: concrete slipway

Suits: dinghies and powered craft

Availability: approx. 2 hours either side HW

Restrictions: speed limit in harbour: water-skiing permitted outside harbour

Facilities: fuel nearby, limited parking (c), toilets, diving supplies and outboard repairs nearby, chandlers in town

Dues: none

Charge: none

Directions: from Glasgow take A82 north then A85 west, following signs in town to car ferries: site is at south side of town at end of railway pier

Waters accessed: Oban Bay and Scottish West Coast

Oban - Port Beag Slip

Tel: (01631) 566088 (Puffin Dive Centre)

Type: wide steep concrete slipway

Suits: powered craft only

Availability: approx. 5 hours either side HW

Restrictions: slip may be blocked in winter by laid-up boats; water-skiing allowed outside harbour

Facilities: fuel nearby, parking for car and trailer (1/2 mile), chandlery in town

Dues: none

Charge: none

Directions: from Glasgow take A82 north then A85 west to Oban and follow Gallanach Rd: site is west of south pier

Waters accessed: Oban Bay and Scottish West Coast

Oban, Gallanach - Port Nan Cuile - (Oban Marine Centre)

Tel: (01631) 562472

Type: shallow concrete ramp

Suits: trailer-sailers and powered craft

Availability: all states of tide

Restrictions: not suitable for sailing dinghies; mainly a diving centre

Facilities:	fuel, parking for car and trailer, toilets, diving supplies and overnight moorings all on site; chandlery and outboard repairs nearby
Dues:	none
Charge:	approx. £5
Directions:	from Oban follow minor road south to Gallanach
Waters accessed:	Sound of Mull, Sound of Kerrera and Scottish West Coast

Ford (Loch Awe)

Type:	concrete slipway
Suits:	all craft
Availability:	at all times
Restrictions:	site is owned by Ford Motor Co and there is locked barrier; obtain key from Ford Motor Hotel: access is via narrow roads
Facilities:	none known
Dues:	none
Charge:	yes
Directions:	from Lochgilphead take A816 north, turning onto B840: site is at southern end of Loch Awe
Waters accessed:	Loch Awe - no access to open sea

Oban, Lerags (Loch Feochan) - Ardoran Marine
Tel: (01631) 566123

Type:	concrete slipway onto mud below half-tide
Suits:	all craft up to 30'/9m LOA except pwc
Availability:	approx. 3 hours either side HW 0800-1800 by prior arrangement
Restrictions:	speed limit: no water-skiing or pwc; access is via single track road
Facilities:	diesel on site, petrol nearby, parking for car and trailer, toilets, limited chandlery, moorings, outboard repairs, cranage and storage on site, diving supplies nearby
Dues:	none
Charge:	approx. £10
Directions:	from Oban follow A816 south for 2 miles, turning off onto minor road to Lerags
Waters accessed:	Loch Feochan, Firth of Lorn and Scottish West Coast

Balvicar (Isle of Seil) - Balvicar Boatyard
Tel: (01852) 300557

Type:	launch small craft from hard or by hoist for larger craft
Suits:	all craft up to 50'/15m and 30 tons
Availability:	approx. 4-5 hours either side of HW by prior arrangement only
Restrictions:	yard work has priority and slip may be blocked - telephone for availability; water-skiing allowed away from moorings

Facilities:	fuel nearby, parking for car and trailer, winter storage, moorings, hoist and all yard facilties on site: toilets, chandlery, diving supplies and engine repairs all available nearby
Dues:	none
Charge:	approx. £10-15 for self-launching
Directions:	from Oban follow A816 south then B844 for 7 miles, turning left at Balvicar village stores
Waters accessed:	Seil Sound, Loch Melfort and Scottish West Coast

Kilmelford (Loch Melfort) - Kilmelford Yacht Haven

Tel: (01852) 200248

Type:	concrete slipway or shingle hard
Suits:	all craft up to 45'/13m LOA
Availability:	all states of tide mon to sat 0830-1700 or at other times by prior arrangement
Restrictions:	check with boatyard before use
Facilities:	diesel, parking for car and trailer, toilets, travel hoist and full boatyard facilities
Dues:	none
Charge:	only if hoist used
Directions:	from Oban take A816 south for 16 miles
Waters accessed:	Loch Melfort and Scottish West Coast

Kilmelford (Loch Melfort) - Melfort Pier and Harbour

Tel: (01852) 200333

Type:	three concrete slipways
Suits:	all craft up to 25'/7.6m LOA
Availability:	approx. 1 hour either side HW by prior arrangement
Restrictions:	access is via narrow single-track road
Facilities:	diesel on site, petrol nearby, limited parking for car and trailer (c), toilets & showers, launderette, engine repairs, dinghy storage, moorings, water, electricity, accommodation, restaurant and bar
Dues:	yes
Charge:	approx. £12
Directions:	from Oban take A816 south to Kilmelford then turn right onto single track Degnish road for 1½ miles; site is at head of Loch Melfort
Waters accessed:	Loch Melfort and Scottish West Coast

Craobh Haven (Loch Shuna) - Craobh Marina

Tel: (01852) 500222 Fax: (01852) 500252

Type:	concrete slipway with hoist for larger craft and shingle hard
Suits:	all craft up to 45'/13m LOA
Availability:	approx. 2 hours either side HW
Restrictions:	5 mph speed limit in harbour: no water-skiing

Facilities:	diesel on site, parking for car and trailer (c), toilets & showers, launderette, engine repairs, water, electricity, chandlery, restaurant and bar
Dues:	none
Charge:	yes
Directions:	from Oban take A816 south towards Lochgilphead
Waters accessed:	Loch Shuna and Scottish West Coast

Ardfern (Loch Craignish) - Ardfern Yacht Centre
Tel: (01852) 500247/500636 Fax: (01852) 500624

Type:	concrete ramp
Suits:	all craft up to 25'/7.6m LOA
Availability:	approx. 3-4 hours either side HW during working hours (0830-1730) by prior arrangement
Restrictions:	5 mph speed limit in marina
Facilities:	diesel on site, parking for car and trailer (c), toilets & showers, water, electricity, moorings, chandlery, repairs and all yard facilities, bar and restaurant
Dues:	none
Charge:	approx. £14 including car parking
Directions:	from Oban follow A816 south, turning onto B8002 for 1 mile: site is at head of Loch Craignish
Waters accessed:	Loch Craignish, Sound of Jura and Scottish West Coast

Crinan (Loch Crinan) - Crinan Ferry

Type:	stone slipway
Suits:	all craft up to 30'/9m LOA
Availability:	approx. 2-3 hours either side HW
Restrictions:	none known
Facilities:	fuel, parking for car and trailer, toilets, chandler nearby: larger craft can be launched by Crinan Boats Ltd Tel: (01546) 830232 for information
Dues:	none known
Charge:	none
Directions:	from Oban follow A816 south, turn onto B8025 south of Kilmartin then right at 'T' junction onto B841: site is old ferry ramp at end of Crinan Canal near Crinan Hotel
Waters accessed:	Loch Crinan

Tayvallich (Loch Sween)

Type:	hard foreshore
Suits:	all craft
Availability:	all states of tide
Restrictions:	none known
Facilities:	none known
Dues:	none
Charge:	none

Directions: from Oban follow A816 south, turning onto B8025 south of Kilmartin then right at 'T' junction onto B841 and left onto B8025: site is on west shore of loch and access is via narrow roads

Waters accessed: Loch Sween, Sound of Jura and Scottish West Coast

Ardrishaig (Crinan Canal) - Pier Square Slipway
Tel: (01546) 603210 (Canal Office)

Type:	steep concrete ramp
Suits:	all craft up to 18'/5.5m LOA
Availability:	approx. 3 hours either side HW 0900-1700 by prior arrangement
Restrictions:	4 knot speed limit in canal: BW Boat Safety Scheme applies to craft using canal; water-skiing permitted in Loch Fyne; permission to use must be obtained - site is used by boatyard; narrow access
Facilities:	fuel in cans nearby, limited parking for car and trailer nearby, toilets, chandlery and outboard repairs nearby
Dues:	approx. £7.50
Charge:	none
Directions:	from Lochgilphead follow A83 south: site is adjacent to main pier near canal sea lock
Waters accessed:	Crinan Canal, Loch Fyne, and Scottish West Coast

Tarbert (East Loch Tarbert) - Pier Road
Tel: (01880) 820376 (TYC Secretary: Ian MacGillvray)

Type:	concrete slipway onto shingle
Suits:	all craft up to 25'/7.6m LOA
Availability:	all states of tide
Restrictions:	4 knot speed limit in harbour: water-skiing permitted outside harbour
Facilities:	fuel and parking for car and trailer nearby (c), toilets; chandlery, diving supplies and outboard repairs in Tarbert
Dues:	none
Charge:	approx. £1
Directions:	from Lochgilphead follow A83 south: site is on south side of harbour in Pier Road adjacent Tarbert Yacht Club
Waters accessed:	East Loch Tarbert, Loch Fyne and Scottish West Coast

Campbeltown Harbour - New Quay Slip, Hall Street
Tel: (01586) 552552 (Harbour Master)

Type:	shallow and wide concrete slipway onto clay/mud
Suits:	all craft up to 30'/9m LOA
Availability:	approx. 3 hours either side HW
Restrictions:	5 mph speed limit in Inner Harbour: water-skiing permitted at Harbour Master's discretion
Facilities:	fuel, parking for car and trailer, toilets, chandlery and outboard repairs all nearby

Dues:	none
Charge:	none
Directions:	from Lochgilphead follow A83 south: site is at head of New Quay and is visible from main roundabout at approach to harbour area
Waters accessed:	Campbeltown Loch, Firth of Clyde and Scottish West Coast

Isle of Arran, Lamlash - Harbour Slipway

Type:	concrete slipway
Suits:	all craft up to 25'/7.6m LOA
Availability:	approx. 3 hours either side HW
Restrictions:	none known
Facilities:	fuel, parking for car and trailer, toilets, chandlery
Dues:	none
Charge:	none
Directions:	from Glasgow follow A738 or A737 south, then A78 north to Ardrossan, ferry to Brodick then A841 south: site is on harbour front
Waters accessed:	Firth of Clyde and Scottish West Coast

Isle of Arran, Whiting Bay - Shore Road

Type:	concrete slipway
Suits:	dinghies only
Availability:	approx. 2½ hours either side HW
Restrictions:	none known
Facilities:	fuel, parking for car and trailer, toilets, chandlery
Dues:	none
Charge:	none
Directions:	from Glasgow follow A738 or A737 south, then A78 north to Ardrossan, ferry to Brodick then A841 south: site is adjacent to pier
Waters accessed:	Firth of Clyde and Scottish West Coast

Crarae (Loch Fyne) - Quarry Point Visitor Centre

Type:	launching over shingle
Suits:	all craft up to 20'/6.1m LOA
Availability:	approx. 3 hours either side HW 1000-1800 Apr to Oct
Restrictions:	none known
Facilities:	fuel, parking for car and trailer, toilets, restaurant and children's facilities
Dues:	none
Charge:	none
Directions:	from Glasgow follow A82 then A83 west to west side of Loch Fyne: site is 2 miles south of Furnace
Waters accessed:	Loch Fyne and Scottish West Coast

St Catherines (Loch Fyne) - St Catherine's Slip

Type:	concrete slipway
Suits:	all craft up to 12'/3.6m LOA
Availability:	approx. 4 hours either side HW
Restrictions:	site mainly used by hotel visitors
Facilities:	parking for car and trailer, other facilities at nearby hotel
Dues:	none
Charge:	none
Directions:	from Glasgow follow A82 then A83 west, taking A815 along east shore of Loch Fyne: site is opposite St Catherine's Hotel
Waters accessed:	Loch Fyne and Scottish West Coast

Tighnabruaich (Kyles of Bute) - Maramarine Ltd, Rhubaan Boatyard
Tel: (01436) 810971

Type:	concrete slipway
Suits:	all craft
Availability:	all states of tide by prior arrangement
Restrictions:	none known
Facilities:	fuel nearby, parking for car and trailer, toilets and boat park on site, chandlery and outboard repairs nearby
Dues:	none
Charge:	none
Directions:	from Glasgow follow A82 then A83 west, taking A815, A886 and A8003 south or ferry to Dunoon A815 then B836 right onto A886 and take A8003 south
Waters accessed:	Kyles of Bute, Loch Riddon and Scottish West Coast

Kames, by Tighnabruaich (Kyles of Bute) - Tank Landing Slip
Tel: (01700) 811632 (Kilfinan Community Council)

Type:	large shallow to moderate concrete slipway
Suits:	all craft up to 25'/7.6m LOA
Availability:	approx. 5 hours either side of HW
Restrictions:	access via narrow single track roads
Facilities:	fuel from garage (2 miles), parking for car and trailer in large car park adjacent, toilets (1 mile), shops; limited chandlery and boat and engine repairs from Tighnabruaich
Dues:	none
Charge:	none
Directions:	from Glasgow follow A82 then A83 west, taking A815, A886 and A8003 south or ferry to Dunoon and A815, then B836 right onto A886 and take A8003 south to Tighnabruaich then follow Shore Rd to Kames keeping left and following signs to Ardlamont: site is 1 mile from Kames crossroads
Waters accessed:	Kyles of Bute, Loch Riddon and Scottish West Coast

Colintraive (Kyles of Bute) - Ferry Stage
Tel: (01700) 841235 (Caledonian Mac Brayne)

Type:	concrete slipway
Suits:	all craft
Availability:	approx. 4 hours either side HW with prior permission only
Restrictions:	ferry must not be obstructed
Facilities:	limited parking for car and trailer, toilets
Dues:	none
Charge:	none
Directions:	from Glasgow take ferry to Dunoon from Gourock and follow A815 and B836 turning left onto A886 south: site is at ferry crossing to Isle of Bute
Waters accessed:	Kyles of Bute, Loch Riddon and Scottish West Coast

Isle of Bute, Rothesay - Outer Harbour Slipway

Type:	concrete slipway
Suits:	all craft
Availability:	approx. 3 hours either side HW
Restrictions:	none known
Facilities:	fuel nearby, parking for car and trailer
Dues:	none
Charge:	none
Directions:	from Glasgow take ferry to Dunoon from Gourock then follow A815 and B836, then left onto A886 south to Colintraive ferry to Isle of Bute, then A886 south to Rothesay; from Inverclyde via Wemyss Bay ferry
Waters accessed:	Kyles of Bute, Loch Riddon and Scottish West Coast

Isle of Bute, Port Bannatyne

Type:	concrete ramp at head of bay
Suits:	all craft up to 25'/7.6m LOA
Availability:	all states of tide
Restrictions:	none known
Facilities:	fuel nearby, parking for car and trailer
Dues:	none
Charge:	none
Directions:	from Glasgow take ferry to Dunoon from Gourock then follow A815 then B836, then left onto A886 south to Colintraive ferry to Isle of Bute then A886 south; from Inverclyde via Wemyss Bay ferry
Waters accessed:	Kyles of Bute, Loch Riddon and Scottish West Coast

Isle of Bute, Port Bannatyne - The Port Yard

Type:	concrete slipway with rails
Suits:	all craft
Availability:	approx. 5 hours either side HW
Restrictions:	none known
Facilities:	fuel, parking for car and trailer (c), crane, winch, toilets, chandlery, repairs, moorings

Dues:	none
Charge:	yes
Directions:	from Glasgow ferry to Dunoon from Gourock follow A815 then B836 left onto A886 south to Colintraive ferry to Isle of Bute then A886 south, or from Inverclyde via Wemyss Bay ferry
Waters accessed:	Kyles of Bute, Loch Riddon and Scottish West Coast

Dunoon (Firth of Clyde) - Port Riddell Slipway, East Bay

Type:	concrete slipway
Suits:	all craft
Availability:	all states of tide
Restrictions:	none known
Facilities:	fuel nearby, limited parking for car and trailer, toilets nearby
Dues:	none
Charge:	not known
Directions:	from Glasgow by ferry from Gourock
Waters accessed:	Firth of Clyde and Scottish West Coast

Sandbank (Holy Loch) - Holy Loch Marina, Rankin's Brae
Tel: (01369) 701800 Fax: (01369) 704749

Type:	concrete slipway
Suits:	all craft
Availability:	approx. 5 hours either side HW by prior arrangement
Restrictions:	4 knot speed limit in marina
Facilities:	fuel, parking for car and trailer, toilets and showers, chandlery and other marina facilities, 23 tonne boat lift
Dues:	no additional charge
Charge:	approx. £10
Directions:	from Glasgow by Gourock ferry to Dunoon and follow A815 north
Waters accessed:	Holy Loch, Firth of Clyde and Scottish West Coast

Clynder (Gare Loch) - Public Slipway, Shore Road

Type:	wide concrete slipway
Suits:	dinghies and power boats
Availability:	all states of tide
Restrictions:	12 mph speed limit,
Facilities:	fuel, parking for car and trailer, toilets, chandlery, diving supplies, outboard repairs nearby, cafe, shop, moorings, boat hire and accomodation: site is adjacent Modern Charters Ltd.
Dues:	none
Charge:	none
Directions:	from Glasgow take A82 onto A814 at Dumbarton to Garelochhead then B833 south to Clynder: site is on west side of loch
Waters accessed:	Gare Loch, Firth of Clyde and Scottish West Coast

Helensburgh (Gare Loch) - Rhu Marina

Tel: (01436) 820238 Fax: (01436) 821039

Type:	launching by travel hoist only
Suits:	larger craft
Availability:	approx. 3 hours either side HW during working hours by prior arrangement
Restrictions:	8 knot speed limit: water-skiing prohibited
Facilities:	diesel, parking for car and trailer, toilets & showers, chandlery and engine repairs all on site
Dues:	marina fees
Charge:	approx. £25 + vat each way
Directions:	from Glasgow take A82 onto A814 at Dumbarton to eastern shore of Gare Loch
Waters accessed:	Gare Loch, Firth of Clyde and Scottish West Coast

Helensburgh (Gare Loch) - Pier

Type:	concrete slipway
Suits:	all craft
Availability:	approx. 3 hours either side HW
Restrictions:	none known
Facilities:	fuel nearby, parking for car and trailer, toilets
Dues:	none
Charge:	yes
Directions:	from Glasgow take A82 onto A814 at Dumbarton and turn left at traffic lights in centre of town: site is adjacent pier
Waters accessed:	Gare Loch, Firth of Clyde and Scottish West Coast

Dumbarton (River Leven) - Bridge Street

Tel: (01389) 737000 (Harbour Master/Director of Roads)

Type:	concrete slipway
Suits:	all craft up to 10'/3m wide
Availability:	approx. 3 hours either side HW
Restrictions:	water-skiing prohibited: River Leven is fast-flowing
Facilities:	fuel nearby, parking for car and trailer on site is often congested, toilets, chandlery and outboard repairs nearby
Dues:	none
Charge:	none
Directions:	from Glasgow follow A82 then A814 into Dumbarton, turn left into High St and then into Bridge St: in Bridge St, take 1st turning on right before crossing bridge and then turn left; site is between two road bridges; no access upstream to Loch Lomond
Waters accessed:	River Leven, Firth of Clyde and Scottish West Coast

Balloch (Loch Lomond) - Loch Lomond Marina, Riverside
Tel: (01389) 752069 Fax: (01389) 753118

Type:	wooden slipway
Suits:	powered craft
Availability:	0900-1900 (summer),0900-1700 (winter) or by prior arrangement
Restrictions:	5 mph speed limit on river but none on loch
Facilities:	fuel (100m), parking for car and trailer (c), toilets & showers, chandlery, outboard repairs and tractor all on site
Dues:	none
Charge:	approx. £10
Directions:	from Glasgow follow A82 north to Balloch, at southern end of Loch Lomond
Waters accessed:	Loch Lomond

Ardlui (Loch Lomond) - Ardlui Marina
Tel: (01301) 704243

Type:	steep concrete ramp onto sandy foreshore
Suits:	all craft except pwc
Availability:	0900-1800
Restrictions:	5 mph speed limit in mooring area: max. width 16'/5m
Facilities:	fuel, parking for car and trailer (c), toilets, berths, boatyard facilities, storage, crane (14 tonne), shop, restaurant, hotel, camping
Dues:	none
Charge:	approx. £10
Directions:	from Erskine Bridge follow A82 north towards Ardlui: site is 8 miles north of Tarbert at north end of Loch Lomond
Waters accessed:	Loch Lomond

Renfrew (River Clyde) - Clyde River Boatyard
Tel: (01418) 865974 Fax: (01418) 863111

Type:	concrete slipway
Suits:	all craft up to 45'/13m LOA and 14 tons max
Availability:	approx. 2½ hours either side HW
Restrictions:	7 knot speed limit in estuary: water-skiing prohibited
Facilities:	diesel on site, petrol 1½ miles, parking for car and trailer (c), toilets, crane and hoist
Dues:	none
Charge:	self-launching approx. £15
Directions:	leave M8 at junction 27 and follow signs to Renfrew: access is via Old Kings Inch Rd
Waters accessed:	Firth of Clyde

Glasgow (Strathclyde Loch) - Strathclyde Country Park, Hamilton

Tel: (01698) 266155

Type:	concrete slipway into 8'/2.4m water
Suits:	dinghies and powered craft
Availability:	0930-dusk daily
Restrictions:	water-skiing permitted in designated area: boat drivers must hold Grade 3 B.W.S.F. licence: all users must report to Booking Office before launching
Facilities:	fuel nearby, parking for car and trailer on site, changing rooms and showers at Water Sports Centre
Dues:	none
Charge:	approx. £2.70 adult & £1.55 juvenile for canoe or sailing dinghy: approx. £16 for speedboat
Directions:	from M74 leave at junction 4 or 5 and follow signs
Waters accessed:	Strathclyde Loch

Port Glasgow (River Clyde) - Coronation Park, East Bay

Tel: (07747) 006755 (Steve Eagin, Parks Dept.)

Type:	concrete slipway
Suits:	all craft up to 25'/7.6m LOA
Availability:	all states of tide except LWS
Restrictions:	none known
Facilities:	fuel (200m), parking for car and trailer, toilets, chandlery and yard facilities nearby
Dues:	none
Charge:	none
Directions:	from M8 follow A8 west: access is via tarred road in park
Waters accessed:	River Clyde and Scottish West Coast

Newark (River Clyde) - Newark Castle Park

Tel: (07747) 006755 (Steve Eagin, Parks Dept.)

Type:	concrete slipway
Suits:	all craft up to 20'/6.1m LOA
Availability:	HW only
Restrictions:	none known
Facilities:	fuel, parking for car only
Dues:	none
Charge:	none
Directions:	follow M8 and A8 west from Glasgow, turning off at Newark roundabout
Waters accessed:	River Clyde and Scottish West Coast

Greenock (River Clyde) - Battery Park

Tel: (07747) 006755 (Steve Eagin, Parks Dept.)

Type:	concrete slipway onto shingle
Suits:	all craft up to 25'/7.6m LOA
Availability:	approx. 2 hours either side HW 0800-1630
Restrictions:	permission to launch required

Facilities:	fuel, parking for car and trailer, toilets, chandlery from Gourock
Dues:	none
Charge:	none
Directions:	follow M8 and A8 west from Glasgow to Greenock: access is from Eldon St into park
Waters accessed:	River Clyde and Scottish West Coast

Gourock (River Clyde) - Cove Road Slipway, Cardwell Bay

Tel: (07747) 006755 (Steve Eagin, Parks Dept.)

Type:	narrow concrete slipway
Suits:	dinghies only
Availability:	approx. 2 hours either side HW
Restrictions:	access is down narrow no-through road
Facilities:	fuel, no parking, chandlery from Gourock
Dues:	none
Charge:	none
Directions:	follow M8 then A8 west to Gourock turning right into Cove Rd
Waters accessed:	River Clyde and Scottish West Coast

Gourock (River Clyde) - Ashton Slipway

Tel: (07747) 006755 (Steve Eagin, Parks Dept.)

Type:	concrete slipway
Suits:	dinghies only
Availability:	approx. 2 hours either side HW
Restrictions:	narrow entrance to site
Facilities:	no fuel, parking, toilets, chandlery from Gourock
Dues:	none
Charge:	none
Directions:	from Glasgow follow M8 then A8 west to Gourock and signs to Ashton: site is on east side of RGYC
Waters accessed:	River Clyde and Scottish West Coast

Gourock (River Clyde) - Maybank Slipway

Tel: (07747) 006755 (Steve Eagin, Parks Dept.)

Type:	concrete slipway
Suits:	dinghies only
Availability:	approx. 2 hours either side HW
Restrictions:	narrow entrance to site
Facilities:	parking in main road only, toilets, chandlery from Gourock
Dues:	none
Charge:	none
Directions:	from Glasgow follow M8 then A8 west to Gourock and signs to Ashton
Waters accessed:	River Clyde and Scottish West Coast

Inverkip (Firth of Clyde) - Kip Marina
Tel: (01475) 521485 Fax: (01475) 521298

Type:	shallow concrete ramp
Suits:	all craft
Availability:	all states of tide during daylight hours by prior arrangement
Restrictions:	3 knot speed limit
Facilities:	diesel on site, petrol nearby, parking for car and trailer, toilets & showers, sauna, chandlery, diving supplies, engine repairs, crane & travel hoist, launderette, bar and restaurant all on site
Dues:	approx. £10
Charge:	approx. £10
Directions:	from Glasgow follow M8 to Greenock then A78 to Inverkip/Wemyss Bay
Waters accessed:	Firth of Clyde, Kyles of Bute and Crinan Canal to Scottish West Coast

Largs (Firth of Clyde) - Barrfields Slipway, North Bay

Type:	concrete slipway
Suits:	all craft up to 18'/5.5m LOA
Availability:	approx. 4 hours either side HW
Restrictions:	slipway must be kept clear at all times for Lifeboat use
Facilities:	fuel nearby, parking for car and trailer nearby, toilets
Dues:	none
Charge:	none
Directions:	from Irvine follow A78 north: access to site is via Shore Rd
Waters accessed:	Firth of Clyde and Scottish West Coast

Largs (Firth of Clyde) - Largs Yacht Haven, Irvine Road
Tel: (01475) 675333

Type:	stone slipway
Suits:	all craft up to 25'/7.6m LOA
Availability:	approx. 3 hours either side HW
Restrictions:	some within marina area: launching difficult in strong SW winds
Facilities:	fuel, parking for car and trailer (c), toilets, chandlery, diving supplies, outboard repairs, travel hoist, bar, restaurant all on site
Dues:	none
Charge:	none
Directions:	from Irvine follow A78 north: site is on left just before railway line off public car park
Waters accessed:	Firth of Clyde, Kyles of Bute and Scottish West Coast

Great Cumbrae Island - Scottish National Watersports Training Centre
Tel: (01475) 674666

Type:	concrete slipway
Suits:	all craft
Availability:	approx. 4 hours either side HW by prior arrangement
Restrictions:	none
Facilities:	fuel from local garage, parking for car and trailer nearby (c), toilets (400m), chandlery in Millport, accommodation
Dues:	none
Charge:	none
Directions:	from Largs by ferry to Great Cumbrae Island: site is on north east corner of island close to ferry terminal
Waters accessed:	Firth of Clyde, Kyles of Bute and Scottish West Coast

Ardrossan (Firth of Clyde) - Clyde Marina, The Harbour
Tel: (01294) 607077 Fax: (01294) 607076

Type:	launching by boat hoist or mobile crane into marina
Suits:	larger craft (20'/6.1m to 100'/30m)
Availability:	during business hours 0900-1800
Restrictions:	5 mph speed limit in marina
Facilities:	diesel on site, petrol nearby, parking for car and trailer, toilets and chandlery and all marina facilities on site; diving supplies and outboard repairs nearby
Dues:	approx. £6.35
Charge:	approx. £60 + vat
Directions:	located near town centre of Ardrossan, approx, 1 hour SW of Glasgow
Waters accessed:	Firth of Clyde, Kyles of Bute and Scottish West Coast

Saltcoats (Firth of Clyde) - Harbour Slipway

Type:	stone ramp
Suits:	all craft
Availability:	approx. 2 hours either side HW
Restrictions:	none known
Facilities:	petrol, parking for car and trailer, toilets nearby
Dues:	none
Charge:	none
Directions:	from Irvine follow A78 north and turn off to Saltcoats
Waters accessed:	Firth of Clyde and Scottish West Coast

Irvine (Firth of Clyde) - Harbour Street Slipway

Type:	concrete slipway
Suits:	all craft up to 18'/5.5m LOA
Availability:	approx. 3 hours either side HW
Restrictions:	launching by arrangement only
Facilities:	parking for car and trailer, toilets nearby; Scottish Maritime Museum
Dues:	none
Charge:	none
Directions:	from Glasgow follow A737 and A736 south: site is in Harbour St close to the Scottish Maritime Museum
Waters accessed:	Firth of Clyde and Scottish West Coast

Troon (Firth of Clyde) - Troon Yacht Haven, The Harbour

Tel: (01292) 315553

Type:	fairly steep (1:8) concrete slipway
Suits:	all craft up to 40'/12.2m LOA except pwc
Availability:	all states of tide
Restrictions:	5 knot speed limit in marina
Facilities:	diesel on site, petrol nearby, parking for car and trailer, toilets & showers, sauna, chandlery, boat and engine repairs, bar and restaurant, tractor assistance if required
Dues:	none
Charge:	approx. £3.50
Directions:	from Glasgow follow A77 south then A78 north and follow signs to Troon: access to site is via Harbour Rd
Waters accessed:	Firth of Clyde and Scottish West Coast

Ayr - South Harbour Street

Tel: (01292) 281687

Type:	steep concrete slipway with vertical drop at end
Suits:	all craft up to 20'/6.1m LOA
Availability:	approx. 4 hours either side HW
Restrictions:	5 knot speed limit in harbour: water-skiing permitted offshore; access may be temporarily restricted by building work
Facilities:	parking for car and trailer nearby
Dues:	none
Charge:	none
Directions:	from Glasgow follow A77 south and from town centre drive down south side of harbour
Waters accessed:	Ayr Bay, Firth of Clyde and Scottish West Coast

Ayr - Ayr Yacht and Cruising Club, South Harbour Street
Tel: (01292) 267963 (Secretary: Miss E. Hope)

Type:	concrete slipway onto gravel
Suits:	all craft
Availability:	4 hours either side HW for larger craft, otherwise all states of tide
Restrictions:	advance notice required and 3rd party indemnity needed; water-skiing permitted offshore
Facilities:	fuel in town, parking for car and trailer (c), toilets, showers, chandlery nearby
Dues:	£5
Charge:	yes
Directions:	from Glasgow follow A77 south to Ayr: from town centre drive down south side of harbour
Waters accessed:	Ayr Bay, Firth of Clyde and Scottish West Coast

Girvan - Harbour Slipway
Tel: (01465) 713648 (Harbour Master)

Type:	steep concrete slipway
Suits:	all craft up to 30'/9m LOA
Availability:	approx. 4 hours either side HW by arrangement with Harbour Master
Restrictions:	4 knot speed limit in harbour: narrow access road
Facilities:	fuel, parking for car and trailer, toilets & showers on site, pontoon berths, chandlery nearby
Dues:	none
Charge:	none
Directions:	from Glasgow follow A77 south, turn off into Newton Place via the Newton Kennedy Bridge: site is on N side of harbour
Waters accessed:	Firth of Clyde and Scottish West Coast

Cairnryan (Loch Ryan) - Cairnryan Slipway

Type:	steep concrete slipway onto shingle
Suits:	small craft only
Availability:	all states of tide
Restrictions:	none known
Facilities:	fuel, parking for car and trailer, toilets
Dues:	none
Charge:	none
Directions:	from Stranraer follow A77 north along east shore of Loch Ryan: site is in picnic area just north of Cairnryan
Waters accessed:	Loch Ryan and Scottish West Coast

Stranraer (Loch Ryan) - Stranraer Harbour
Tel: (01776) 702460 (Harbour Master)

Type:	shallow concrete slipway
Suits:	all craft
Availability:	approx. 2 hours either side HW
Restrictions:	none known
Facilities:	fuel, parking for car and trailer (c), toilets, chandlery, outboad repairs all nearby
Dues:	approx. £3.70
Charge:	none
Directions:	from Dumfries follow A75 west to Stranraer: site is behind Ulster Bus Depot at southernmost point of Loch Ryan between Sea Containers and Stena Line
Waters accessed:	Loch Ryan and Scottish West Coast

Wig Bay (Loch Ryan) - Wig Bay Slip

Type:	concrete slipway
Suits:	all craft
Availability:	all states of tide
Restrictions:	permission to launch should be obtained from Loch Ryan S.C.
Facilities:	fuel, parking for car and trailer
Dues:	none
Charge:	none
Directions:	from Dumfries follow A75 west then A718 north: site is on west shore Loch Ryan south of Kirkcolm Pt and adjacent Loch Ryan S.C.
Waters accessed:	Loch Ryan and Scottish West Coast

Lady Bay (Loch Ryan)

Type:	concrete slipway onto sand
Suits:	small craft only
Availability:	all states of tide
Restrictions:	site is private but free access is normally granted
Facilities:	parking for car and trailer, picnic area
Dues:	none
Charge:	none
Directions:	from Dumfries follow A75 west then A718 north: site is on west shore Loch Ryan
Waters accessed:	Loch Ryan and Scottish West Coast

Portpatrick - Harbour Slipway

Type:	concrete slipway onto shingle and soft sand
Suits:	dinghies only
Availability:	approx. 2 hours either side HW
Restrictions:	consult Harbour Master before use; access is steep, narrow and partially obstructed
Facilities:	fuel, parking for car and trailer, toilets
Dues:	none

Charge:	none
Directions:	from Stranraer follow A716 south then A77 west: site is on south side of Outer Harbour near disused lighthouse
Waters accessed:	North Channel and Scottish West Coast

Port Logan

Type:	concrete slipway onto sand
Suits:	small craft only
Availability:	all states of tide
Restrictions:	none known
Facilities:	parking for car and trailer, toilets
Dues:	none
Charge:	none
Directions:	from Stranraer follow A716 south then B7065 to Port Logan
Waters accessed:	Port Logan Bay and Scottish West Coast

Mull of Galloway

Type:	slipway of granite and stone blocks
Suits:	all craft
Availability:	approx. 2 hours either side HW
Restrictions:	site is private but free access is normally given: there are very strong tides in the vicinity of up to 6 knots on spring tides
Facilities:	parking for car and trailer
Dues:	none
Charge:	none
Directions:	from Stranraer follow A716 south then B7041 and narrow track to Mull Lighthouse
Waters accessed:	Luce Bay, North Channel and Scottish West Coast

Drummore Harbour

Type:	steep concrete slipway onto hard sand
Suits:	dinghies only
Availability:	approx. 2 hours either side HW
Restrictions:	padlocked gate: key held at Ship Inn; there are very strong tides in the bay on spring tides
Facilities:	fuel, parking for car and trailer (c), toilets; Kirkmaiden B.C. is nearby
Dues:	none
Charge:	none
Directions:	from Stranraer follow A716 south to W side of Luce Bay: access is directly from road at bottom of village and opposite Ship Inn
Waters accessed:	Luce Bay and Scottish West Coast

Sandhead

Type:	launching over soft sand
Suits:	small craft
Availability:	all states of tide
Restrictions:	watch out for nearby bombing range signals
Facilities:	fuel, parking for car and trailer, toilets
Dues:	none
Charge:	none
Directions:	from Stranraer follow A716 south: site is on west shore Luce Bay
Waters accessed:	Luce Bay and Scottish West Coast

Port William

Tel: (01988) 700464 (J.Brawls) or 0402 488255

Type:	shallow and narrow concrete ramp onto gravel beach
Suits:	small craft only
Availability:	approx. 2 hours either side HW
Restrictions:	narrow road and tight bend at top of slip
Facilities:	toilets on site, fuel, parking for car and trailer and outboard repairs nearby
Dues:	approx. £3.70
Charge:	none
Directions:	from Newton Stewart take A714 south to Wigtown, then A714 to Port William
Waters accessed:	Luce Bay and Scottish West Coast

Isle of Whithorn - Harbour Slipway

Tel: (01988) 500468 (S. McGuire, Harbour Master)

Type:	medium concrete slipway onto sand/mud
Suits:	all craft
Availability:	approx. 3 hours either side HW
Restrictions:	5 mph speed limit: consult Harbour Master before use
Facilities:	fuel, parking for car and trailer, toilets, winch, water, electricity, hotel/restaurant, toilets, chandlers and outboard repairs
Dues:	approx. £4.35
Charge:	none
Directions:	from Stranraer follow A75 then A747 south: from Dumfries, follow A75 west to Newton Stewart, then turn south for Isle of Whithorn
Waters accessed:	Wigtown Bay, Solway Firth and Scottish West Coast

Garlieston - Harbour

Tel: (01988) 600274/ 600259

Type:	shallow concrete ramp
Suits:	all craft
Availability:	approx. 3 hours either side HW
Restrictions:	contact Harbour Master before launching
Facilities:	fuel nearby, parking for car and trailer on site; toilets, chandlery, fresh water, electricity, outboard repairs,

	moorings all nearby
Dues:	approx. £4.35 inc. vat
Charge:	none
Directions:	from Dumfries follow A75 east to Newton Stewart then take A714 south turning onto B7004 1 mile south of Kirkinner: site is on west side of bay in sheltered harbour
Waters accessed:	Wigtown Bay and Scottish West Coast

Borgue (Dee Estuary) - Brighouse Bay Holiday Park
Tel: (01557) 870267

Type:	concrete slipway
Suits:	all craft
Availability:	most states of tide - difficult at LWS
Restrictions:	obtain permission from park reception prior to launching
Facilities:	parking for car and trailer, toilets, shop, leisure club, golf course and indoor swimming pool all on site
Dues:	included in fee
Charge:	approx. £7.50 weekdays and £10 weekends
Directions:	from Kirkcudbright follow A755 west for ½ mile, turning left onto B727 signposted Borgue: after 4 miles take left turning signposted Brighouse Bay: site is on right after 2 miles
Waters accessed:	Dee Estuary and North Irish Sea

Kirkcudbright (Dee Estuary) - Harbour Slipway
Tel: (01557) 331135 (Harbour Master)

Type:	uneven stone slipway onto shingle
Suits:	all craft up to 15'/4.6m LOA except speedboats
Availability:	approx. 2 hours either side HW
Restrictions:	5 mph speed limit: water-skiing and pwc prohibited, contact the Harbour Master prior to launching
Facilities:	fuel from garage, parking for car and trailer in car park, toilets, chandlery, diving supplies, outboard repairs and pontoon berths
Dues:	none
Charge:	none
Directions:	from Dumfries follow A75 west for approx. 15 miles, then turn left onto A711: site is on east shore of estuary
Waters accessed:	Dee Estuary and North Irish Sea

Kippford (Solway Firth)

Type:	concrete slipway onto shingle
Suits:	all craft up to 18'/5.5m LOA
Availability:	approx. 2 hours either side HW
Restrictions:	none known
Facilities:	fuel, parking for car and trailer, toilets, chandlery
Dues:	none
Charge:	none
Directions:	from Dumfries follow A711 to Dalbeattie then A710 south for 4 miles turning right onto minor road
Waters accessed:	Solway Firth and North Irish Sea

Parton (Loch Ken) - Galloway Sailing Centre

Tel: (01644) 420626

Type:	shallow concrete slipway
Suits:	all craft up to 28'/8.5m LOA except pwc
Availability:	0900-1900 Easter to end Oct
Restrictions:	10 mph speed limit: pwc prohibited; 3rd party insurance certificate required
Facilities:	fuel (3 miles), parking for car and trailer, toilets & showers, changing rooms, chandlery; outboard repairs nearby
Dues:	none
Charge:	approx. £7
Directions:	from Dumfries follow A75 to Castle Douglas then north onto A713: site is 10 miles north and is clearly signposted on left-hand side beyond Parton
Waters accessed:	Loch Ken only

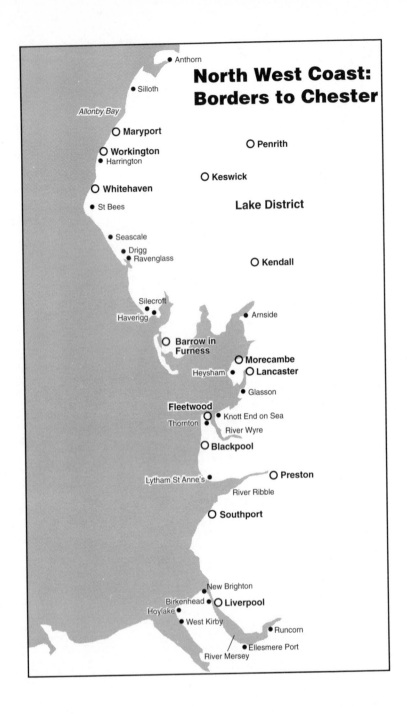

North West Coast: Borders to Chester

Anthorn (Solway Firth) - Foreshore

Type:	launching over shingle foreshore
Suits:	light craft which can be manhandled
Availability:	approx. 2 hours either side HW
Restrictions:	site suitable for dinghies only
Facilities:	fuel from garage, parking for car and trailer
Dues:	none
Charge:	none
Directions:	from Carlisle follow B5307 to Kirkbride then minor roads north for 4 miles
Waters accessed:	Solway Firth

Silloth (Solway Firth) - Promenade Slipway
Tel: (01900) 326333 (Borough of Allerdale)

Type:	steep concrete ramp onto shingle/mud foreshore
Suits:	small sailing and powered craft
Availability:	approx. 2 hours either side HW
Restrictions:	water-skiing permitted but site is exposed: RNLI inshore rescue boat has priority use at all times
Facilities:	fuel in town, parking for car and trailer and toilets on site; outboard repairs and other facilties in town
Dues:	none
Charge:	none
Directions:	from Carlisle follow A595/6 south, turning off onto B5302: access to site, which is next to the lifeboat station, is from the Promenade
Waters accessed:	Solway Firth

Allonby Bay (Solway Firth)
Tel: (016973) 22620 (Solway Rural Iniative)

Type:	shallow concrete ramp onto shingle/mud foreshore with some boulders
Suits:	dinghies and small powered craft
Availability:	approx. 2 hours either side HW
Restrictions:	water-skiing permitted but site is exposed: narrow access to car park; site is in Solway Coast AONB- do not disturb wildlife - contact number above for further advice
Facilities:	fuel from Maryport, parking for car and trailer and toilets on site, other facilities in Maryport
Dues:	none
Charge:	none
Directions:	from Maryport follow B5300 north for approx. 5 miles: site is just north of village and access is through car park
Waters accessed:	Solway Firth

Maryport (Solway Firth) - Maryport Marina, Marine Road

Tel: (01900) 814431

Type:	shallow concrete ramp (1:12)
Suits:	all craft except pwc and windsurfers
Availability:	approx. 2½ hours either side HW by prior arrangement
Restrictions:	4 knot speed limit in harbour: water-skiing allowed offshore
Facilities:	diesel on site, petrol nearby, parking for car and trailer, toilets, chandlery and outboard repairs all on site
Dues:	none
Charge:	approx. £10 (inc. parking)
Directions:	from Carlisle follow A596 south; in Maryport, follow Stenhouse Street, turning left into Irish Street then right into Marine Road
Waters accessed:	Solway Firth

Workington (Solway Firth) - Tidal Dock

Tel: (01946) 831696 (Vanguard Sailing Club)

Type:	concrete slipway
Suits:	all craft up to 35'/10.7m LOA
Availability:	approx. 2½ hours either side HW, or later for small craft
Restrictions:	slow speed in harbour: water-skiing allowed to seaward of Lifeboat mooring
Facilities:	fuel in town (1 mile), parking for car and trailer; associate membership of club with use of facilities available
Dues:	not known
Charge:	approx. £3
Directions:	from Carlisle follow A596 south; site is on south side of dock just seaward of railway bridge
Waters accessed:	Solway Firth

Harrington (Solway Firth) - Harbour Slipway

Tel: (01946) 830600 (Harrington Sailing & Fishing Club)

Type:	concrete slipway
Suits:	trailer-sailers
Availability:	approx. 2 hours either side HW
Restrictions:	permission to use slipway must be obtained in advance; this is a small port, giving access to exposed open sea conditions, which is not suitable for dinghies and inflatables
Facilities:	fuel, parking for car and trailer, toilets
Dues:	not known
Charge:	yes
Directions:	from Workington follow A597 south for approx. 3 miles
Waters accessed:	Solway Firth

Whitehaven (Solway Firth) - West Pier Slipway
Tel: (01946) 692435 (Harbour Office, Duke Street)

Type:	fairly steep stone slipway
Suits:	all craft except pwc
Availability:	approx 3 hours either side HW
Restrictions:	8 knot speed limit in harbour: site has locked barrier; this is a busy fishing harbour and prior permission to use slipway must be obtained from the Harbour Master
Facilities:	diesel on site, petrol, parking for car and trailer (c), toilets and outboard repairs all nearby
Dues:	no separate fee
Charge:	approx. £5
Directions:	follow A595 to town centre and follow signs from Market Place to West Pier
Waters accessed:	Solway Firth and Irish Sea

Whitehaven (Solway Firth) - Custom House Quay Slipway
Tel: (01946) 692435 (Harbour Office, Duke Street)

Type:	fairly steep concrete slipway
Suits:	all craft except pwc and windsurfers
Availability:	at all times into locked Inner Harbour
Restrictions:	8 knot speed limit in harbour: access to Outer Harbour and sea is via sealock; for permission to enter lock call "Whitehaven Harbour" on VHF Ch12 or telephone (01946) 694672
Facilities:	diesel on site, petrol, parking for car and trailer (c), toilets and outboard repairs all nearby
Dues:	no separate fee
Charge:	approx. £5
Directions:	follow A595 to town centre: site is close to Market Place
Waters accessed:	Solway Firth and Irish Sea

St Bees - Main Beach

Type:	concrete slipway (1:11)
Suits:	small craft only
Availability:	approx. 2 hours either side HW or at all times over beach
Restrictions:	site is very exposed in onshore winds: once craft is launched, vehicle must be returned to car park and the lifeboat must not be obstructed
Facilities:	fuel nearby, parking for car and trailer and toilets on site
Dues:	none
Charge:	none
Directions:	from Whitehaven follow B5345 south to St Bees and local roads to beach
Waters accessed:	Irish Sea

St Bees - Seamill

Type:	concrete ramp
Suits:	small craft only
Availability:	approx. 2 hours either side HW or at all states of tide over beach
Restrictions:	site is very exposed in onshore winds
Facilities:	diesel nearby, parking for car and trailer and toilets on site
Dues:	none
Charge:	none
Directions:	from Whitehaven follow B5345 south to St Bees, following main street to Seamill, at south end of beach
Waters accessed:	Irish Sea

Seascale - Beach

Type:	launching over shingle beach
Suits:	light craft
Availability:	all states of tide in offshore winds only
Restrictions:	site is very exposed in onshore winds
Facilities:	parking for car and trailer
Dues:	none
Charge:	none
Directions:	from Whitehaven follow A595 south turning onto B5344
Waters accessed:	Irish Sea

Drigg - Beach

Type:	launching over pebble and sand beach
Suits:	light craft
Availability:	at HW in offshore winds only
Restrictions:	site is very exposed and dangerous in onshore winds
Facilities:	parking for car and trailer
Dues:	none
Charge:	none
Directions:	from Whitehaven follow A595 south to Holmrook and turn onto B5344; follow minor roads over railway line to shore (approx. 1 mile)
Waters accessed:	Irish Sea

Ravenglass

Type:	concrete ramp or over beaches into harbour
Suits:	all craft
Availability:	approx. 2 hours either side HW
Restrictions:	harbour is very exposed and dangerous in onshore winds and currents within the harbour are very strong
Facilities:	fuel from garage, parking for car and trailer nearby, pub and shop
Dues:	none

Charge:	none
Directions:	follow A595 south turning off into village; site is at end of street into natural harbour formed by the rivers Irt, Mite and Esk
Waters accessed:	Irish Sea

Silecroft - Beach

Type:	launching over steep shingle bank and pebble and sand beach: 4-wheel drive vehicle or tractor tow is essential
Suits:	small craft
Availability:	near HW in offshore winds only
Restrictions:	site is very exposed and dangerous in onshore winds
Facilities:	diesel nearby, parking for car and trailer, toilets and water on site: site is used by South Cumbria Sea Angling Club
Dues:	none
Charge:	none
Directions:	from Whitehaven follow A595 south turning onto the minor road which leads off at the junction of A595 and A5093; site is in car park at end of road
Waters accessed:	Irish Sea

Haverigg

Type:	concrete slipway
Suits:	small craft only
Availability:	approx. 2½ hours either side HW
Restrictions:	not known
Facilities:	parking for car and trailer
Dues:	none
Charge:	none
Directions:	from Whitehaven follow A595 and A5093 south to Millom turning onto minor roads to Haverigg: site is at mouth of Duddon Estuary close to Rugby Union Club
Waters accessed:	Duddon Estuary and Irish Sea

Barrow-in-Furness - The Promenade, Isle of Walney
Tel: (01229) 894784 Tourist Information Centre

Type:	wide stone slipway
Suits:	all craft
Availability:	at all states of tide
Restrictions:	none
Facilities:	fuel from garage (1 mile), parking for car and trailer nearby
Dues:	none
Charge:	none
Directions:	from Barrow in Furness follow A590 onto the island; site is opposite the Ferry Hotel
Waters accessed:	Irish Sea

Barrow-in-Furness - The Causeway, Roa Island
Tel: (01229) 894784 (Tourist Information Centre)

Type:	concrete slipway
Suits:	small craft
Availability:	at all states of tide across beach
Restrictions:	none
Facilities:	fuel from garage (1 mile), parking for car and trailer on road
Dues:	none
Charge:	none
Directions:	from Barrow-in-Furness follow A5087 and minor road onto the causeway, turning off to beach
Waters accessed:	Irish Sea

Arnside (Kent estuary) - Promenade

Type:	concrete slipway onto soft mud
Suits:	all craft
Availability:	all states of tide
Restrictions:	beware of strong tide and the 'bore' in the Kent Estuary
Facilities:	fuel, parking for car and trailer (c), toilets in village; visitors are welcome at the Arnside S.C. on promontory at end of Promenade
Dues:	none
Charge:	none
Directions:	leave M6 at junction 36 taking A590 north and then left onto B5282: site is adjacent Crossfields Boatyard at seaward end of Promenade
Waters accessed:	Kent Estuary, Morecambe Bay and Irish Sea

Morecambe - Promenade
Tel: (01524) 582808 (Tourist Information Centre)

Type:	4 shallow concrete slipways onto shingle, two near Town Hall, two at Green Street
Suits:	all craft; powercraft discouraged Sept - May
Availability:	approx. 3 hours either side HW
Restrictions:	8 mph speed limit inshore: water-skiing, windsurfing and pwc permitted outside 200m; obtain permit for vehicular access to Promenade; Promenade Supervisor on duty all year and lifeguards in summer; this is a major conservation area
Facilities:	fuel nearby, parking for car in Marine Drive or nearby car parks (c), trailers may be left near slipways for up to 24 hrs, toilets and other facilities nearby; tractor available for boat recovery from Dinghy Angling Club; RNLI station at Green Street
Dues:	none
Charge:	none
Directions:	leave M6 at junction 33 / 34 through Lancaster or junction 35 via Carnforth: sites are located on 5 mile stretch of Promenade
Waters accessed:	Morecambe Bay and Irish Sea

Glasson Dock (Lune Estuary) - Glasson Basin Yacht Co

Tel: (01524) 751491

Type:	concrete slipway into locked basin
Suits:	larger craft
Availability:	by prior arrangement only
Restrictions:	24 hrs notice required to lock out into Glasson Dock - gates can be opened 1 hour before HW: access to Lancaster Canal is via locks
Facilities:	fuel, parking for car and trailer (c), toilets & showers, chandlery, crane, winch and other boatyard facilities
Dues:	BW licence required if entering canal network
Charge:	approx. £2.50 per metre each way
Directions:	turn off A6 between Garstang and Lancaster to follow signs to Glasson Dock
Waters accessed:	Lancaster Canal and River Lune Estuary via Glasson Dock

Glasson Dock (Lune Estuary) - Glasson S.C., Fishnet Point

Tel: (01524) 751089

Type:	concrete ramp
Suits:	all craft up to 20'/6.1m LOA
Availability:	approx. 1½ hours either side HW
Restrictions:	dinghy racing has priority over all other uses
Facilities:	fuel nearby, parking for car and trailer, toilets & showers, bar & winch on site, other facilities nearby
Dues:	none
Charge:	approx. £10
Directions:	turn off A6 between Garstang and Lancaster to follow signs to Glasson Dock
Waters accessed:	River Lune Estuary, Morecambe Bay and Irish Sea

Knott-End-on-Sea (River Wyre) - Knott End Ferry Stage

Tel: (01253) 771175 (Swift Offshore Services)

Type:	wide, shallow concrete ramp
Suits:	all craft: pwc welcome
Availability:	at all time at neaps but approx. 4 hours either side HW at Springs
Restrictions:	ferries must not be obstructed
Facilities:	fuel nearby, parking for car and trailer on site, toilets nearby
Dues:	not known
Charge:	approx. £8 (£58.75 p.a.) for boats and £5 for pwc
Directions:	turn off M55 to Blackpool onto A585 and follow signs: site is at ferry terminal opposite Fleetwood
Waters accessed:	River Wyre and Irish Sea

Thornton (River Wyre) - Stanah Car Park
Tel: (01253) 891000 (Wyre Borough Council)

Type:	fairly steep concrete slipway (1:10)
Suits:	all craft up to 25'/7.6m LOA
Availability:	approx. 2 hours either side HW
Restrictions:	none known
Facilities:	parking for car and trailer, toilets
Dues:	none known
Charge:	none
Directions:	leave M55 at junction 3 taking A585 towards Fleetwood, turning right into Skippool Rd then right again into River Rd
Waters accessed:	River Wyre and Irish Sea

Thornton (River Wyre) - Skippool Creek, Wyre Road
Tel: (01253) 891000 (Wyre Borough Council)

Type:	small shallow concrete ramp
Suits:	sailing dinghies and canoes: no pwc
Availability:	approx. 1 hour either side HW
Restrictions:	access road is tidal: reckless navigation is prohibited; slipway is liable to mud siltation
Facilities:	fuel nearby, parking for car and trailer nearby
Dues:	none
Charge:	none
Directions:	from M55 follow A585 for Fleetwood: at large round-about by River Wyre Hotel turn right and take first right again, following signposts to Skippool Creek
Waters accessed:	River Wyre Estuary

Blackpool - Little Bispham, Princes Way
Tel: (01253) 626141 (Chief Beach Patrol Officer)

Type:	concrete ramp onto sand and shingle beach
Suits:	small craft
Availability:	all states of tide if suitable vehicle is used
Restrictions:	8 knot speed limit within 200m LWS mark
Facilities:	parking for car and trailer in car park(c) and toilets nearby
Dues:	none
Charge:	none
Directions:	from M55 follow signs to seafront: from Blackpool Tower, continue along the Promenade northwards for approx. 3 1/2 miles, turning left for site at Little Bispham tramstop
Waters accessed:	Irish Sea

Blackpool - Starr Gate

Tel: (01253) 626141 (Chief Beach Patrol Officer)

Type:	concrete ramp onto sand and shingle beach
Suits:	small craft
Availability:	all states of tide if suitable vehicle is used
Restrictions:	8 knot speed limit within 200m LWS mark
Facilities:	parking for car and trailer in car park (c) and toilets on site
Dues:	none
Charge:	none
Directions:	from M55 follow signs to seafront: from Blackpool Tower, continue along the Promenade southwards for approx. 3 miles and site is on right
Waters accessed:	Irish Sea

Lytham St Anne's (Ribble Estuary) - Lytham Boat Yard, Dock Road

Tel: (01253) 795307

Type:	concrete slipway
Suits:	all craft
Availability:	approx. 2 hours either side HW
Restrictions:	speed limit; water-skiing permitted in river
Facilities:	fuel, parking for car and trailer, toilets & showers, limited chandlery, water, electricity and other boatyard facilities
Dues:	none
Charge:	approx. £5
Directions:	from M55 turn off at junction 4 and take A583 south, then minor roads: access to site is via Dock Rd
Waters accessed:	Ribble Estuary and Irish Sea

Lytham St Anne's - Fairhaven Lake

Tel: (01253) 735439 (Fylde Borough Council)

Type:	launching from grass bank
Suits:	sailing dinghies, windsurfers, canoes and rowing boats
Availability:	at all times (non-tidal)
Restrictions:	no powered craft
Facilities:	parking for car and trailer (c), restaurant, picnic area
Dues:	yes
Charge:	yes
Directions:	follow A584 1½ miles south from Lytham St Anne's
Waters accessed:	Fairhaven Lake only

Preston - Douglas Boatyard, Becconsall Lane, Hesketh Bank

Tel: (01772) 812462

Type:	concrete slipway
Suits:	larger sailing and motor cruisers from 20'/6.1m - 50'/15m LOA
Availability:	approx. 2 hours either side of HW by prior arrangement
Restrictions:	speed limit near moorings
Facilities:	diesel on site, petrol nearby, parking for car and trailer, toilets, chandlery, moorings and yard services all on site
Dues:	on application
Charge:	on application
Directions:	from Preston take A59 south to Tarleton turning onto road towards Hesketh Bank: take first right after Becconsall Hotel into Becconsall Lane
Waters accessed:	Rivers Douglas and Ribble and the Irish Sea

Liverpool Docks- Salthouse Slipway, Salthouse Dock

Tel: (0151) 709 6558 (Harbour Master)

Type:	steep concrete slipway (1:8) into 12'/3.7m water in dock complex
Suits:	small craft
Availability:	0900-sunset by prior arrangement
Restrictions:	licence required before launching: speed limit; no water-skiing; site gives access to approx. 65 acres of water but with restricted headroom under bridges
Facilities:	fuel nearby, parking for car and trailer on site (c), toilets, chandlery, watersports centre, shops and restaurants all available nearby
Dues:	licence required
Charge:	approx. £5.50
Directions:	from M62 follow signs to Liverpool City Centre / Pier Head / Albert Dock, turning off Inner Ring Road to Albert Dock
Waters accessed:	South Docks: access to River Mersey by prior arrangement

Liverpool Docks - Liverpool Marina, Coburg Wharf, Sefton St

Tel: (0151) 708 5228

Type:	large shallow concrete ramp into locked basin
Suits:	all craft except pwc and windsurfers
Availability:	0900-1730 by prior arrangement
Restrictions:	5 knot speed limit: access to tidal river through Brunswick Dock lock gates which open approx. 2$\frac{1}{2}$ hours either side HW (end March-end Oct) or by arrangement
Facilities:	diesel on site, petrol nearby, parking for car and trailer (c), toilets & showers, chandlery and other marina facilities on site
Dues:	approx. £15

Charge:	no additional fee
Directions:	from Inner Ring Rd follow signs to Albert Dock Complex: marina is in Coburg Dock off Sefton St to south of Albert Dock
Waters accessed:	Dock complex and River Mersey via lock

New Brighton (Mersey Estuary) - South Slipway, Victoria Road
Tel: (0151) 647 2366 (Metropolitan Borough of Wirral)

Type:	concrete slipway onto hard sand
Suits:	all craft
Availability:	at all states of tide except 1 hour either side LWS during daylight hours
Restrictions:	8 knot speed limit inshore on North Wirral coast: this is a major shipping river with strong currents and pleasure craft must obey Port Regulations: site is very busy at weekends in summer; barrier may be locked when Warden is on site
Facilities:	fuel from nearby garage, parking for car and trailer nearby (with permit), toilets on Promenade, chandlery and outboard repairs nearby
Dues:	yes
Charge:	yes: permit is required for vehicles driving on foreshore - contact number above
Directions:	leave M53 at junction 1 and follow signs to seafront: site lies at the eastern end of the Promenade
Waters accessed:	Mersey Estuary

Hoylake (Mersey Estuary) - Dove Point Slipway, Meols
Tel: (0151) 647 2366 (Metropolitan Borough of Wirral)

Type:	concrete slipway onto hard sand
Suits:	sailing craft: no pwc
Availability:	approx. 2 hours either side HW
Restrictions:	8 knot speed limit inshore on North Wirral coast: pwc prohibited; locked barrier when staff on site
Facilities:	fuel from nearby garage, parking for car on Promenade and for trailer by slipway, toilets and chandlery nearby
Dues:	none
Charge:	none, but permit is required for vehicles driving on foreshore - contact number above
Directions:	leave M53 at junction 2 taking A551/A553: site is at the eastern end of the Meols Promenade by the Coastguard Office
Waters accessed:	Mersey Estuary and Irish Sea

West Kirby (West Kirby Marine Lake) - Sandy Lane Slipway
Tel: (0151) 647 2366 (Metropolitan Borough of Wirral)

Type:	shallow concrete ramp onto foreshore
Suits:	all craft except pwc
Availability:	approx. 2½ hours either side HW
Restrictions:	pwc prohibited
Facilities:	fuel in West Kirby, parking for car and trailer on Promenade, toilets, chandlery and outboard repairs nearby
Dues:	none
Charge:	none but permit is required - contact number above
Directions:	leave M53 at junction 2 following A551/A553: site is at southern end of the West Kirby Marine Lake which is well signposted
Waters accessed:	Dee Estuary and Irish Sea

LAKE DISTRICT

Coniston Water

The lake is approx. 5 miles/8 km long: small non-powered craft may be launched from public access land but powered craft can only be launched from Coniston Boating Centre; there is a speed limit of 10 mph on the lake.

Coniston - Coniston Boating Centre, Lake Road
Tel: (015394) 41366 (Lake District National Park Authority)

Type:	steep concrete ramp
Suits:	all craft up to 26'/7.9m LOA except pwc
Availability:	0900-1730 daily
Restrictions:	10 mph speed limit: narrow bridge on approach road to site; this is the only launching site for powered craft on the lake
Facilities:	fuel nearby, parking for car and trailer on site, toilets, cafe, picnic area, boat park; hand-winch and 4-wheel drive assistance available (c); chandlers in Windermere, outboard repairs in Kendall
Dues:	none
Charge:	approx. £8.50
Directions:	from M6 turn off at junction 36 and take A590/A591 to Windermere, continuing to Ambleside and turning onto A593 to Coniston: turn left by garage into Lake Rd
Waters accessed:	Coniston Water

Coniston - Monk Coniston Car Park
Tel: (015394) 41533 (Tourist Information Centre)

Type:	launching over gravel shore
Suits:	small non-powered craft only
Availability:	during daylight hours
Restrictions:	powered craft prohibited
Facilities:	fuel in Coniston, parking for car and trailer (c) and toilets on site
Dues:	none
Charge:	none
Directions:	leave M6 at junction 36 and take A590/A591 to Windermere, continuing to Ambleside and turning onto A593 to Coniston: turn left onto B5285 following road round north shore of lake; site is reached through car park
Waters accessed:	Coniston Water

Coniston - Brown Howe Car Park
Tel: (015394) 41533 (Tourist Information Centre)

Type:	launching over gravel shore
Suits:	small non-powered craft only
Availability:	during daylight hours
Restrictions:	powered craft prohibited

Facilities:	fuel nearby, parking for car and trailer on site (c), toilets on site
Dues:	none
Charge:	none
Directions:	leave M6 at junction 36 and take A590/A591 to Windermere, continuing to Ambleside; turn onto A593 to south of Coniston taking the A5084 to SW corner of lake: site is reached through car park
Waters accessed:	Coniston Water

Derwentwater

There is a 10 mph speed limit on the lake

Keswick - Keswick-on-Derwentwater Launch Co Ltd

Tel: (017687) 72263

Type:	launching over shingle shore
Suits:	small craft only
Availability:	0900-2130 (Mar-Nov)
Restrictions:	10 mph speed limit on lake
Facilities:	parking for car and trailer, toilets
Dues:	none
Charge:	approx. £3.50
Directions:	leave M6 at junction 40 and follow A66 west to Keswick: site is on west shore of lake
Waters accessed:	Derwentwater

Portinscale, Keswick - Derwentwater Marina

Tel: (017687) 72912

Type:	2 concrete ramps into 3'/1m water
Suits:	all craft up to 25'/7.6m LOA and 10'/3m wide
Availability:	during daylight hours
Restrictions:	10 mph speed limit on lake
Facilities:	fuel from Keswick, parking for car and trailer, toilets and showers, picnic area, chandlery, outboard repairs. bar and restaurant
Dues:	none
Charge:	approx. £6
Directions:	leave M6 at junction 40 following A66 west to Keswick and continuing on to Portinscale; turn left after crossing river and site is ½ mile after village
Waters accessed:	Derwentwater

Portinscale, Keswick - Nichol End Marine

Tel: (017687) 73082

Type:	steel slipway into 4'/1.2m water
Suits:	all craft up to 25'/7.6m LOA except pwc
Availability:	at all times, preferably by prior arrangement
Restrictions:	10 mph speed limit on lake

Facilities:	diesel nearby, petrol, parking for car and trailer, toilets & showers, chandlery, outboard repairs, boat repairs, refreshments, tuition and boat hire all on site
Dues:	none
Charge:	approx. £6.50 (inc. overnight mooring if required)
Directions:	leave M6 at junction 40 following A66 west to Keswick and continuing on to Portinscale; turn left following brown signs for 1/2 mile through village
Waters accessed:	Derwentwater

Derwentwater - Kettlewell Car Park

Tel: (01768) 774649 (National Trust)

Type:	launching over shingle foreshore
Suits:	small non-powered craft only
Availability:	during daylight hours
Restrictions:	10 mph speed limit: powered craft prohibited; site is conservation area
Facilities:	limited parking for car and trailer on site (c), toilets in Lodore
Dues:	none
Charge:	none
Directions:	leave M6 at junction 40 and follow A66 west to Keswick; turn left onto Borrowdale road (B5289) and follow for approx. 21/2 miles: site is 1/2 mile north of Lodore
Waters accessed:	Derwentwater

Ullswater

The lake is approx. 8 miles/13 kms long and 1 km at its widest point. There is a 10 mph speed limit on the lake: the National Trust do not permit the launching of powered craft from their land.

Ullswater - Glencoyne Bay

Tel: (017684) 82067 (National Trust)

Type:	launching over gravel foreshore
Suits:	small non-powered craft only
Availability:	during daylight hours: telephone to notify intentions
Restrictions:	10 mph speed limit: powered craft prohibited; craft must be manhandled across road from car park
Facilities:	limited parking for car and trailer on site (c), toilets nearby
Dues:	none
Charge:	none
Directions:	leave M6 at junction 40 and follow A66 west, turning left onto A592 and following road to Glencoyne: site is close to bridge
Waters accessed:	Ullswater

Ullswater - Howtown

Tel: (017684) 86530/82414 (Tourist Information Centre, Easter - Oct.)

Type:	steep hardcore ramp
Suits:	craft up to 20'/6.1m LOA
Availability:	during daylight hours
Restrictions:	10 mph speed limit: narrow no-through road
Facilities:	fuel and toilets nearby, very limited parking on site
Dues:	none
Charge:	none
Directions:	leave M6 at junction 40 and follow A66 west turning left onto A592; at top of lake turn left onto B5320 to Pooley Bridge and follow minor road south for 3 miles
Waters accessed:	Ullswater

Ullswater - The Spit, Glenridding (Glenridding Sailing Centre)

Tel: (017684) 82541

Type:	launching over shingle foreshore
Suits:	sailing dinghies, windsurfers and canoes
Availability:	1000-1700 daily (end Mar-Oct)
Restrictions:	10 mph speed limit: all launchers must report to office on arrival: personal buoyancy must be worn: launching is at site owners' discretion; locked barrier at night
Facilities:	parking for car and trailer on site, toilets nearby, safety boats
Dues:	none
Charge:	approx. £4
Directions:	leave M6 at junction 40 and follow A66 west, turning left onto A592 and following road to Glenridding: access to site is via drive between the Ullswater and Glenridding Hotels and opposite the entrance to National Park Car Park
Waters accessed:	Ullswater

Lake Windermere

This is the largest English lake, at 10½ miles/17km long and 1¼ miles/2 km at its widest point. There are speed limits in some areas of the lake and all powered craft wishing to use the lake must be registered (c) at the Lake Warden's Office at Ferry Nab. The National Trust do not permit launching of powered craft or water-skiing from their shoreline. There are patrol craft on the lake to offer assisitance and to enforce the byelaws - details of which may be obtained from the Lake Warden Tel: (015394) 42753.

Bowness-on-Windermere - Ferry Nab Public Slipway

Tel: (015394) 42753 (Lake Warden's Office)

Type:	concrete ramp into 6'/1.8m water: tractor assistance available (c)
Suits:	craft up to 35'/10.7m LOA and 11 tons max. inc. trailer and vehicle
Availability:	daily 0800-2200 in summer and 0900-1700 in winter

Restrictions:	6 mph speed limit in certain areas: all powered craft must be registered at slipway office; strict regulations for water-skiing (tel. office for details); towed inflatables prohibited
Facilities:	fuel nearby, parking for car and trailer (c), showers and boat park on site, toilets in car park; chandlery and outboard repairs available from boatyards nearby
Dues:	annual registration fee approx £5 p.a. (less than 10hp) or £25 p.a. (10-80hp)
Charge:	approx. £6 if non-powered and £12.50 if powered
Directions:	leave M6 at junction 36 and take A590/A591 to roundabout at N. end of Kendal by-pass; take either the B5284 signposted Hawkshead via ferry or continue to Windermere and turn left onto A592 to Bowness
Waters accessed:	Lake Windermere

Ambleside - Waterhead

Tel: (015394) 42753 (Lake Warden's Office)

Type:	launching over shingle beach
Suits:	craft up to 20'/6.1m LOA and 5hp engine capacity
Availability:	during daylight hours
Restrictions:	6 mph speed limit in certain areas; all powered craft must be registered; strict regulations for water-skiing (ask at office), towed inflatables prohibited
Facilities:	fuel from Waterhead Marine, parking for car and trailer (c), toilets
Dues:	annual registration fee approx £5 p.a.(less than 10hp) or £25 p.a.(10-80hp)
Charge	yes
Directions:	from M6 turn off at junction 36 and take A590/A591 to Windermere, continuing to Ambleside; turn onto A591 south
Waters accessed:	Lake Windermere

Ambleside - Low Wray Campsite

Tel: (015394) 32810 (National Trust Warden)

Type:	launching over gravel shore
Suits:	small non-powered craft only
Availability:	during daylight hours
Restrictions:	powered craft prohibited: facility generally only available for use by campers at site; non-campers should telephone first
Facilities:	parking for car and trailer on site, toilets, other facilities from boatyards nearby
Dues	included in launching fee
Charge	yes
Directions:	leave M6 at junction 36 and take A590/A591 to Windermere, continuing to Ambleside; turn onto B5286 and follow signs: site is 3 miles south of Ambleside
Waters accessed:	Lake Windermere

Harrowslack

Tel: (015394) 44746 (National Trust Warden)

Type:	launching over gravel shore
Suits:	small non-powered craft only
Availability:	during daylight hours
Restrictions:	powered craft prohibited: permit must be obtained from N.T. Warden at Harrowslack House
Facilities:	parking for car and trailer on site
Dues	included in launching fee
Charge	approx. £1
Directions:	leave M6 at junction 36 and take A590/A591 to Windermere, continuing to Ambleside; turn onto B5286 and then follow B5285 from Hawkshead; site is on NW shore of lake
Waters accessed:	Lake Windermere

Newby Bridge - Fell Foot Park

Tel: (015395) 31273 (Park Manager)

Type:	medium concrete ramp
Suits:	sailing craft up to 25'/7.6m LOA and small powered craft up to 5hp
Availability:	0900-1700 by prior arrangement; gates locked at 1900 or dusk if earlier
Restrictions:	6 mph speed limit in certain areas: open speedboats over 5hp and pwc prohibited: cruisers with engines but with separate lockable living accomodation are allowed
Facilities:	fuel from garage in Newby Bridge (2 miles), parking for car and trailer, toilets and cafe available on site: jetty space available by prior arrangement
Dues	none
Charge	approx. £9 inc. parking
Directions:	turn off M6 at junction 36 taking A590 to Newby Bridge and then A592: site is after 1 mile on left at south end of lake on east shore; please use north entrance
Waters accessed:	Lake Windermere

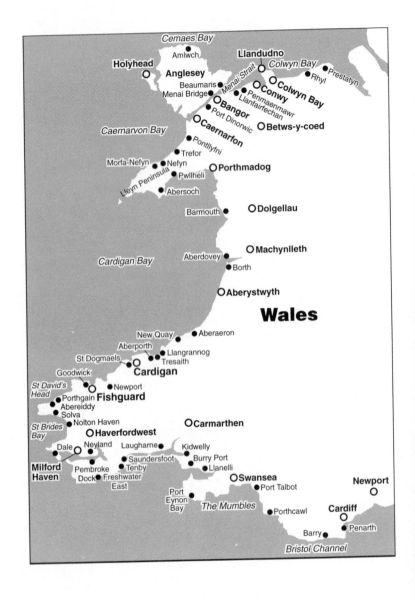

Prestatyn - Slipway

Tel: (01824) 706000 (Denbighshire Council)

Type:	concrete ramp onto firm sandy beach
Suits:	all craft with 4-wheel drive vehicle or tractor
Availability:	approx. 3-4 hours either side HW
Restrictions:	site is base of Prestatyn S.C.: (7'/2.1m) height restriction in car park
Facilities:	parking for car and trailer (c), tractor launch (c) and temporary membership of club available, hotel adjacent
Dues:	none
Charge:	none
Directions:	follow minor road north from coastal road (A548): site is adjacent Sands Hotel
Waters accessed:	Liverpool Bay

Rhyl - Rhyl Yacht Club, Foryd Harbour

Tel: (01745) 334365

Type:	concrete slipway
Suits:	all craft
Availability:	approx. 2 hours either side HW by prior arrangement
Restrictions:	5 mph speed limit in harbour: water-skiing permitted outside harbour
Facilities:	fuel from garage, parking for car and trailer (c), toilets in clubhouse
Dues:	none
Charge:	yes
Directions:	from Chester follow A55 west, turning onto A525 to Rhyl; in town centre turn left onto A548; site is on south side of bridge
Waters accessed:	Kinmel Bay, Liverpool Bay and Irish Sea

Colwyn Bay - Victoria Pier Slipway

Tel: (01492) 596253 (Harbour Master, Conwy)

Type:	shallow concrete ramp onto sand
Suits:	pwc only
Availability:	all states of tide over beach
Restrictions:	10 knot speed limit inshore: site is for pwc only; max.75 craft allowed; on sun and BH priority is given to members of Colwyn Jet Ski Club
Facilities:	fuel nearby, parking for car and trailer, toilets, chandlery, outboard repairs and cafe all on site
Dues:	none
Charge:	approx. £8.50
Directions:	from Chester follow A55 towards Conwy taking Colwyn Bay exit: follow signs to Promenade and site is by Pier
Waters accessed:	Colwyn Bay and Irish Sea

Colwyn Bay, Rhos-on-Sea - Aberhod Slipway
Tel: (01492) 596253 (Harbour Master, Conwy)

Type:	shallow concrete ramp onto sand
Suits:	small craft which can be manhandled: no pwc
Availability:	all states of tide over beach but best 4 hours either side HW
Restrictions:	10 knot speed limit within 200m of shore with access lane for water-skiing: pwc prohibited; registration and proof of insurance required; site is sheltered and used by local S.C.
Facilities:	fuel nearby, parking for car and trailer, toilets, cafe all on site
Dues:	none
Charge:	approx. £8.50
Directions:	from Chester follow A55 towards Conwy, taking Colwyn Bay exit and following signs to Promenade; site is opposite Aberhod Old Hall Hotel
Waters accessed:	Colwyn Bay and Irish Sea

Conwy Morfa - Beacons Recreational Area
Tel: (01492) 596253 (Harbour Master, Conwy)

Type:	steep concrete slipway
Suits:	all craft
Availability:	approx. 3 hours either side HW
Restrictions:	5 mph speed limit inshore: water-skiing permitted outside harbour
Facilities:	fuel nearby, parking for car and trailer and refreshments on site, toilets, chandlery and outboard repairs nearby
Dues:	none
Charge:	approx. £8.50
Directions:	from Chester follow A55 west through the Conwy Tunnel, taking the exit immediately after the tunnel and following signs to 'Beacons'
Waters accessed:	Conwy Bay and Irish Sea

Penmaenmawr - New Promenade
Tel: (01492) 622321 (Penmaenmawr Y.C.)

Type:	shallow concrete ramp onto hard sand
Suits:	small sailing craft and windsurfers: no powered craft
Availability:	all states of tide over beach by prior arrangement with S.C. only
Restrictions:	10 knot speed limit: powered craft prohibited
Facilities:	fuel nearby, parking for car and trailer and toilets on site
Dues:	none
Charge:	none
Directions:	from Conwy follow A55 expressway and signs to Penmaenmawr: access is via road over expressway at west end of Promenade
Waters accessed:	Conwy Bay, Menai Straits and Irish Sea

Llanfairfechan - Llanfairfechan Sailing Club, The Promenade
Tel: (01248) 680301

Type:	concrete slipway
Suits:	small craft
Availability:	all states of tide over beach
Restrictions:	none
Facilities:	parking for car and trailer (c), toilets in clubhouse, dinghy park, temporary membership available to visitors
Dues:	none
Charge:	yes
Directions:	from Conwy follow A55 expressway and signs to Llanfairfechan: site is on Promenade
Waters accessed:	Conwy Bay, Menai Straits and Irish Sea

Bangor - A M Dickie & Sons, Garth Road
Tel: (01248) 352775

Type:	launching by hoist into dock
Suits:	larger craft
Availability:	by prior arrangement
Restrictions:	telephone for details
Facilities:	fuel, parking for car and trailer (c), chandlery and yard facilties
Dues:	none known
Charge:	on application
Directions:	from Conwy follow A55 expressway, turning onto A4087 to Bangor town centre and follow signs to Garth
Waters accessed:	Menai Straits, Conwy Bay and Irish Sea

Anglesey, Menai Bridge - Porth Wrach
Tel: (01248) 712312 (Harbour Master, Isle of Anglesey County Council)

Type:	broad shallow concrete ramp
Suits:	all craft
Availability:	all states of tide
Restrictions:	tides run very fast here and local advice should be taken before launching; 20'/6.1m height restriction on access
Facilities:	fuel nearby, parking for car and trailer and toilets near-by
Dues:	none
Charge:	none
Directions:	from Conwy follow A55/A5 over bridge turning into Beach Rd then Water Rd
Waters accessed:	Menai Straits, Conwy Bay and Irish Sea

Anglesey, Beaumaris - Gallows Point (ABC Powermarine Ltd.)

Tel: (01248) 811413

Type:	concrete ramp
Suits:	all craft
Availability:	approx. 3 hours either side HW 0900-2000 daily
Restrictions:	8 knot speed limit in moorings
Facilities:	fuel, parking for car and trailer, toilets, chandlery, outboard repairs and storage all on site: tractor and boat hoist also available
Dues:	none
Charge:	approx. £4
Directions:	site is ½ mile before Beaumaris town on the A5025
Waters accessed:	Menai Straits, Conwy Bay and Irish Sea

Anglesey - Traeth Bychan

Type:	shallow concrete ramp onto hard sand
Suits:	small craft which can be manhandled
Availability:	all states of tide across beach
Restrictions:	8 knot speed limit in bay: narrow access road
Facilities:	fuel nearby, parking for car and trailer (c), toilets, shop and cafe on site; chandlery and outboard repairs nearby
Dues:	none
Charge:	none
Directions:	from Menai Bridge follow A5025 for approx. 12 miles north then narrow road to Traeth Bychan, 2 miles north of Benllech
Waters accessed:	Irish Sea

Anglesey, Amlwch - Marine Terminal

Tel: (01407) 831065 (Dockmaster)

Type:	steep concrete slipway in Inner Harbour
Suits:	all craft
Availability:	approx. 2 hours either side HW
Restrictions:	contact Dockmaster before launching: dead slow speed limit in harbour - this is a busy fishing and commercial harbour; narrow access to slipway
Facilities:	fuel and other facilties nearby, parking for car and trailer on site
Dues:	none
Charge:	none
Directions:	from Menai Bridge follow A5025 north
Waters accessed:	Irish Sea

Anglesey, Cemaes Bay - Harbour Slipway

Type:	wide concrete slipway into small drying harbour
Suits:	all craft
Availability:	approx. 2 hours either side HW
Restrictions:	8 knot speed limit inshore: access can be very congested
Facilities:	fuel, parking for car and trailer

Dues:	none
Charge:	none
Directions:	from Menai Bridge follow A5025 north; site is on north coast of Anglesey
Waters accessed:	Irish Sea

Anglesey, Holyhead - Newry Beach
Tel: (01407) 762304 (Harbour Master, Stena Line)

Type:	concrete slipway
Suits:	all craft
Availability:	approx. 3 hours either side HW
Restrictions:	speed limit in harbour: this is a busy ferry port; water-skiing permitted offshore
Facilities:	fuel, parking for car and trailer, chandlery nearby
Dues:	none
Charge:	none
Directions:	from Menai Bridge follow A5 north to Holy Island: site is 100m past Coastguard Station
Waters accessed:	Irish Sea

Anglesey - Treaddur Bay, Holy Island

Type:	concrete ramp onto hard sand foreshore
Suits:	all craft
Availability:	all states of tide
Restrictions:	8 knot speed limit in bay and swim-only area
Facilities:	fuel, parking for car and trailer, toilets, chandlery, diving supplies, shops, cafe all nearby
Dues:	none
Charge:	none
Directions:	follow A5 from Menai Bridge towards Holyhead: turn left onto B4545 at valley traffic lights and continue for 3 miles
Waters accessed:	Caernarfon Bay and Irish Sea

Anglesey, Llanfairpwll - Plas Coch Hotel & Caravan Park
Tel: (01248) 714272/714295

Type:	concrete slipway
Suits:	small craft
Availability:	all states of tide
Restrictions:	use of site by prior arrangement only
Facilities:	parking for car and trailer, toilets and showers
Dues:	none
Charge:	yes
Directions:	follow A55/A5 across Menai Bridge, turning left onto A4080
Waters accessed:	Menai Straits

Plas Menai - Plas Menai National Watersports Centre

Tel: (01248) 670964

Type:	concrete slipway with winch
Suits:	small craft
Availability:	approx. 4 hours either side HW by prior arrangement only
Restrictions:	water-skiing permitted; prior notice is necessary and times are restricted by Centre use; launching is at owner's risk
Facilities:	fuel from garage, parking for car and trailer (c), toilets
Dues:	none
Charge:	yes
Directions:	from Bangor follow A487 west for approx. 4 miles, turning off and following signs
Waters accessed:	Menai Strait

Caernarfon - Victoria Dock Slipway

Tel: (01286) 672118 (Harbour Master, Caernarfon Harbour Trust)

Type:	fairly steep concrete ramp
Suits:	all craft: pwc regulated
Availability:	approx. 3 hours either side HW
Restrictions:	5 knot speed limit in sensitive areas; pwc must be registered with Harbour Office (c), have proof of insurance, behave responsibly and observe Port bye-laws; Caernarfon Harbour Trust will prosecute any flagrant breach of Port bye-laws
Facilities:	fuel from Safeways, parking for car and trailer (c) on Slate Quay or Victoria Dock, toilets on Slate Quay, chandlers and outboard repairs from Victoria Dock
Dues:	none
Charge:	none - but £10 registration fee for pwc
Directions:	follow signs in Caernarfon to harbour: access is through Victoria Dock access road which is congested in summer
Waters accessed:	Menai Strait and Caernarfon Bay

Pontllyfni

Type:	concrete slipway onto shingle and sand
Suits:	craft up to 15'/4.6m LOA
Availability:	all states of tide
Restrictions:	none
Facilities:	fuel, parking for car and trailer
Dues:	none
Charge:	none
Directions:	from Caernarfon follow A487/499 towards Pwllheli: site is adjacent West Point Beach Holiday Camp
Waters accessed:	Caernarfon Bay

Trefor - Harbour Slipway

Type:	concrete slipway
Suits:	small craft
Availability:	approx. 3 hours either side HW
Restrictions:	8 knot speed limit inshore
Facilities:	parking for car and trailer
Dues:	none
Charge:	none
Directions:	from Caernarfon follow A487/499 towards Pwllheli and turn off right to Trefor: site is on Lleyn Peninsular
Waters accessed:	Caernarfon Bay

Nefyn - Beach

Type:	launching over hard shingle beach
Suits:	small craft
Availability:	all states of tide except LWS
Restrictions:	8 knot speed limit inshore: water-skiing permitted in designated area offshore
Facilities:	parking for car and trailer but not on beach
Dues:	none
Charge:	none
Directions:	from Caernarfon follow A487/499 towards Pwllheli, turning onto B4417 at Llanaelhaearn: site is on north coast of Lleyn Peninsula
Waters accessed:	Caernarfon Bay

Morfa-Nefyn - Porth Dinllaen Beach

Type:	launching over hard shingle beach into sheltered north-facing bay
Suits:	small craft
Availability:	all states of tide except LWS
Restrictions:	8 knot speed limit inshore: water-skiing permitted in designated area offshore
Facilities:	parking for car and trailer but not on beach
Dues:	none
Charge:	none
Directions:	from Caernarfon follow A487/499 towards Pwllheli, turning onto B4417 at Llanaelhaearn: site is on north coast of Lleyn Peninsula
Waters accessed:	Caernarfon Bay

Abersoch - Porth Fawr

Type:	concrete slipway
Suits:	small craft
Availability:	all states of tide
Restrictions:	8 knot speed limit inshore; water-skiing permitted off-shore
Facilities:	fuel nearby, parking for car and trailer (c), toilets in car park, chandlery in village

Dues:	none
Charge:	yes
Directions:	from Porthmadog follow A497/A499 west
Waters accessed:	Cardigan Bay

Abersoch - Golf Road Beach Entrance

Type:	concrete slipway onto firm sand
Suits:	all craft up to 20'/6.1m LOA
Availability:	all states of tide 0600-2200
Restrictions:	8 knot speed limit inshore; water-skiing permitted off-shore
Facilities:	fuel nearby, parking for car and trailer, chandlery in village
Dues:	none
Charge:	yes, pay car park attendant
Directions:	from Porthmadog follow A497/A499 to Abersoch village turning into Golf Rd: access to site is through car park
Waters accessed:	Cardigan Bay

Abersoch - Min-y-Don Boatyard
Tel: (01758) 740648 (evenings)

Type:	concrete slipway
Suits:	all craft up to 20'/6.1m LOA
Availability:	all states of tide
Restrictions:	8 knot speed limit inshore; water-skiing permitted in designated area offshore with access lane
Facilities:	fuel nearby, parking for car and trailer, toilets nearby, other facilities in village
Dues:	none
Charge:	approx. £10
Directions:	from Porthmadog follow A497/A499 west to Abersoch: site is at bottom of hill and adjacent to the Lifeboat Station
Waters accessed:	Cardigan Bay and Irish Sea

Pwllheli - Outer Harbour
Tel: (01758) 704081 (Harbour Master 0900-1700, 24hr answerphone)

Type:	steep concrete ramp
Suits:	all craft up to 20'/6.1m LOA
Availability:	at all states of tide
Restrictions:	4 knot speed limit in harbour: water-skiing permitted outside harbour; narrow access road
Facilities:	fuel from marina, parking for car and trailer nearby, toilets, chandlery and other boatyard facilities adjacent
Dues:	none
Charge:	approx. £6.50
Directions:	from Porthmadog follow A497 west into Pwllheli and then head for Gimlet Rock
Waters accessed:	Tremadog Bay, Cardigan Bay and Irish Sea

Pwllheli - Wm Partington Marine Ltd, Outer Harbour
Tel: (01758) 612808

Type:	concrete slipway
Suits:	all craft: winch available for larger craft
Availability:	all states of tide, ask at chandlery shop
Restrictions:	4 knot speed limit in harbour: water-skiing and pwc permitted outside harbour
Facilities:	fuel, parking for car and trailer and toilets nearby, chandlery, storage and repairs on site
Dues:	none
Charge:	approx. £3
Directions:	from town centre follow signs to Gimlet Rock Caravan Site
Waters accessed:	Tremadog Bay, Cardigan Bay and Irish Sea

Pwllheli - Promenade

Type:	concrete ramps onto sandy beach
Suits:	small craft which can be manhandled
Availability:	all states of tide
Restrictions:	8 knot speed limit inshore
Facilities:	fuel nearby, parking for car and trailer, toilets and chandlers nearby
Dues:	none
Charge:	none
Directions:	from Porthmadog follow A497 west
Waters accessed:	North Cardigan Bay and Irish Sea

Cricieth - Cricieth Slipway
Tel: (01766) 512927 (Porthmadog Harbour Master)

Type:	shallow concrete ramp onto shingle foreshore
Suits:	all craft: pwc must be registered
Availability:	approx. 2 hours either side HW
Restrictions:	4 mph speed limit until seaward of yellow beach-markers; no craft allowed in designated safe bathing areas; all pwc must be registered with Harbour Office (c) and show proof of insurance; offshore patrol - bye-laws are strictly enforced
Facilities:	fuel, parking for car and trailer (c) and toilets nearby
Dues:	£10 registration fee for pwc
Charge:	approx. £6.50
Directions:	from Caernarfon follow A 487 to Porthmadog then A497 for 3 miles to Criccieth; slipway is adjacent breakwater and opposite lifeboat station and road access is narrow
Waters accessed:	Tremadog Bay, North Cardigan Bay and Irish Sea

Porthmadog - Black Rock Sands, Morfa Bychan
Tel: (01766) 512927 (Harbour Master)

Type:	launching over shallow sandy beach
Suits:	small sailing and powered craft: pwc must be registered (c)
Availability:	all states of tide
Restrictions:	4 mph speed limit in marked launching lane; all craft excluded from buoyed bathing areas; pwc must be registered and show proof of insurance; beach closed nightly in summer from 2000-0900; site often congested
Facilities:	fuel nearby, parking for car and trailer on beach (c), toilets; beach patrolled by Beach Officers - bye-laws are strictly enforced
Dues:	£10 registration fee for pwc
Charge:	approx. £6.50 for boats and £10 for pwc
Directions:	from Caernarfon take A487 to Porthmadog turning right at Woolworths and following signs for 3 miles to Black Rock Sands
Waters accessed:	Tremadog Bay, North Cardigan Bay and Irish Sea

Porthmadog - Harbour Slipway
Tel: (01766) 512927 (Harbour Office)

Type:	concrete ramp, steep at top and shallow at bottom
Suits:	all craft up to 23'/7m LOA: pwc must be registered (c)
Availability:	approx. 3 hours either side HW
Restrictions:	6 knot speed limit within harbour limit and 4 mph within 100m of shore in other areas: no craft allowed in designated bathing areas; water-skiing permitted outside these limits; pwc must be registered (c) and show proof of insurance; locked barrier controlled by Harbour Master
Facilities:	fuel, parking for car and trailer, toilets, chandlery, outboard repairs, boatyard and most other facilities nearby
Dues:	£10 registration fee for pwc
Charge:	approx. £6.50 for boats and £10 for pwc
Directions:	from the north, take A487 via Caernarfon, turning right after the park then taking first left; from the south, cross embankment and turn left after the pelican crossing
Waters accessed:	Tremadog Bay, North Cardigan Bay and Irish Sea

Porthmadog - Porthmadog Sailing Club, The Tilewharf
Tel: (01766) 513546

Type:	steep concrete slipway with electric winch available
Suits:	sailing dinghies only up to 17'/5.2m LOA (no catamarans)
Availability:	approx. 3 hours either side HW

Restrictions:	6 knot speed limit within harbour limit and 4 mph within 100m shore in other areas; no craft allowed in designated safe bathing areas: temporary membership of club needed
Facilities:	fuel, parking for car and trailer, crane by arrangement, toilets on site, chandlery nearby
Dues:	none
Charge:	yes
Directions:	from Conwy follow A470 turning onto A487: at Pen-y-Cei on west side of harbour turn left and follow narrow road right to end
Waters accessed:	Tremadog Bay, North Cardigan Bay and Irish Sea

Llanbedr, Shell Island

Type:	concrete slipway
Suits:	small craft only
Availability:	approx. 3 hours either side HW
Restrictions:	obtain permission to launch from owners on site
Facilities:	parking for car and trailer, toilets and other facilities on camp site: daily visitors welcome
Dues:	none
Charge:	yes
Directions:	from Harlech follow A496 south; turn onto minor road by church in Llanbedr and follow for approx. 2 miles west: site is across causeway (impassable within 1 hour HW) on privately-owned island
Waters accessed:	Tremadog Bay, Cardigan Bay and Irish Sea

Barmouth (Mawddach Estuary) - Harbour Slipway, The Quay
Tel: (01341) 280671 (Harbour Master)

Type:	steep concrete slipway onto soft sand
Suits:	all craft: pwc must be registered (c)
Availability:	approx. 2½ hours either side HW
Restrictions:	5 knot speed limit in harbour
Facilities:	diesel on site, petrol nearby, parking for car nearby (c), trailers may be left on site, toilets, chandlery and repairs available on site
Dues:	£10 registration fee for pwc
Charge:	approx. £10
Directions:	from Conwy follow A470 to Llaneltyd, turning onto A496: in Barmouth turn left under railway bridge; site is at mouth of estuary
Waters accessed:	Mawddach Estuary, Cardigan Bay and Irish Sea

Tywyn - Warwick Road Slipway
Tel: (01654) 767626 (Aberdyfi Harbour Master)

Type:	steep concrete ramp onto shallow sand foreshore
Suits:	all craft
Availability:	all states of tide by prior arrangement
Restrictions:	4 mph speed limit inshore

Facilities:	fuel nearby, parking for car and trailer and toilets on site, chandlery, diving supplies, outboard repairs, shops and pubs all nearby
Dues:	approx. £10.50
Charge:	no additional fee
Directions:	follow A493 from Machynlleth or Dolgellau
Waters accessed:	Cardigan Bay and Irish Sea

Aberdyfi (Aberdovey) (Dyfi Estuary) - Church Bay Slipway
Tel: (01654) 767626 (Harbour Master)

Type:	medium concrete slipway onto hard-packed shingle and mud
Suits:	all craft up to 19'/5.8m LOA
Availability:	approx. 5 hours either side HW
Restrictions:	4 mph speed limit inshore: water-skiing restricted
Facilities:	fuel nearby, parking for car nearby, trailers may be left on site, toilets, chandlery, outboard repairs, shops and pubs nearby
Dues:	approx. £10.50
Charge:	no additional fee
Directions:	on A493 between Machynlleth (9 miles) and Tywyn (5 miles)
Waters accessed:	Dyfi Estuary, Cardigan Bay and Irish Sea

Aberdyfi (Aberdovey) (Dyfi Estuary) - Dovey Yacht Club
Tel: (01654) 767607 (Clubhouse)

Type:	concrete slipway onto sand
Suits:	dinghies only
Availability:	all states of tide
Restrictions:	5 knot speed limit within moorings: no powered craft allowed: temporary membership of club required - contact Secretary
Facilities:	fuel and parking for car and trailer (1/4 mile) (c), crane , toilets on site; chandlery and repairs nearby
Dues:	none known
Charge:	yes
Directions:	turn off A487 north of Machynlleth onto A493 to Aberdovey
Waters accessed:	Dyfi Estuary, Cardigan Bay and Irish Sea

Borth - Aber Leri Boatyard, Ynyslas
Tel: (01970) 871713

Type:	concrete slipway
Suits:	all craft except pwc
Availability:	approx. 2 1/2 hours either side HW 0800-2100
Restrictions:	4 knot speed limit in moorings: pwc prohibited
Facilities:	diesel nearby, parking for car and trailer (c) on site, toilets, chandlery, repairs and all yard services available on site
Dues:	none

Charge:	approx. £6
Directions:	follow B4572 north through Borth village for 1¼ miles
	past golf course: site is next to the river before the bridge
Waters accessed:	River Leri, River Dyfi, Cardigan Bay and Irish Sea

Borth - Beach Slipway

Tel: (01970) 611433 (Aberystwyth Harbour Master)

Type:	shallow wooden ramp onto hard-packed sand beach
Suits:	small craft
Availability:	all states of tide in calm conditions
Restrictions:	8 knot speed limit within 200m of shore: pwc (stand up) prohibited; site is open to west and launching is not possible in high seas or heavy swell
Facilities:	fuel nearby, parking for car and trailer (c) and toilets on site, chandlery and outboard repairs nearby
Dues:	none
Charge:	approx. £4
Directions:	from Aberystwyth follow A487 north, turning left onto B4572 to Borth
Waters accessed:	Cardigan Bay and Irish Sea

Aberystwyth - Harbour Slipway

Tel: (01970) 611433 (Harbour Master)

Type:	shallow concrete ramp
Suits:	all craft up to 20'/6.1m LOA with < 3'/1m draught
Availability:	approx. 2 hours before HW to 3 hours after HW
Restrictions:	5 knot speed limit within harbour limits and 8 knots within 200m of shore; bar at harbour mouth limits access to -3HW+4 in calm conditions for craft with up to 3'/1m draft
Facilities:	diesel on site, petrol nearby, parking for car and trailer and toilets on site, chandlery and outboard repairs nearby
Dues:	none
Charge:	approx. £4
Directions:	from Cardigan follow A487 north to town centre and then signs to harbour
Waters accessed:	Cardigan Bay and Irish Sea

Aberystwyth - Aberystwyth Marina

Tel: (01970) 611422

Type:	steep concrete ramp
Suits:	all craft except pwc
Availability:	approx. 3 hours either side HW
Restrictions:	5 knot speed limit within harbour limits and 8 knots within 200m of shore: pwc prohibited; bar at harbour limits access to -3HW+4 in calm conditions for craft with up to 3'/1m draft
Facilities:	diesel on site, petrol nearby, parking for car and trailer on site; toilets and outboard repairs nearby

Dues:	none
Charge:	approx. £5
Directions:	from Cardigan follow A487 north to town centre and then signs to harbour
Waters accessed:	Cardigan Bay and Irish Sea

Aberaeron Harbour - South Beach

Tel: (01545) 571645 VHF Ch 14 (Harbour Master)

Type:	shallow concrete ramp into harbour
Suits:	all craft
Availability:	approx. 2½ hours either side HW
Restrictions:	8 knot speed limit within 200m of shore
Facilities:	diesel on site, parking for car and trailer (c) on site, toilets, nearby; Aberaeron Y.C. has bar and showers
Dues:	approx. £7.50
Charge:	no additional fee
Directions:	from Cardigan follow A487 north; access is via South Beach car park, signposted 'Beach' just south of town
Waters accessed:	Cardigan Bay and Irish Sea

New Quay - Harbour Slipway

Tel: (01545) 560368 (Harbour Master)

Type:	steep cobbled slipway onto sandy beach
Suits:	all craft
Availability:	approx. 3 hours either side HW
Restrictions:	3 knot speed limit in harbour, 5 knots in bay and 8 knots off beaches: access to site is via steep one-way street
Facilities:	diesel and toilets on site, limited parking for car and trailer nearby
Dues:	approx. £7.50
Charge:	no additional fee
Directions:	from Cardigan follow A487 north, taking A486 west at Synod Inn; from Aberaeron, follow A487 south, taking B4342 west at Llanarth
Waters accessed:	Cardigan Bay and Irish Sea

Llangranog - Slipway

Type:	concrete slipway
Suits:	dinghies and trailer-sailers
Availability:	approx. 3 hours either side HW
Restrictions:	8 knot speed limit inshore: access to site is via narrow roads
Facilities:	petrol, parking for car and trailer (c)
Dues:	none
Charge:	none
Directions:	from Cardigan follow A487 north to Brynhoffnant, turn left onto B4334
Waters accessed:	Cardigan Bay and Irish Sea

Tresaith - Beach

Type:	launching over shingle beach
Suits:	small craft
Availability:	all states of tide
Restrictions:	8 knot speed limit inshore: access to site is via narrow road
Facilities:	parking for car and trailer (c), toilets
Dues:	none
Charge:	none
Directions:	follow A487 north from Cardigan, turning off onto minor roads at Tan-y-groes
Waters accessed:	Cardigan Bay and Irish Sea

Aberporth - Slipway

Type:	steep concrete slipway
Suits:	dinghies and trailer-sailers
Availability:	approx. 3 hours either side HW
Restrictions:	8 knot speed limit inshore: access to site is via narrow road
Facilities:	petrol, parking for car and trailer (c), toilets
Dues:	none
Charge:	none
Directions:	from Cardigan follow A487 north to Blaenannerch, turn left onto B4333
Waters accessed:	Cardigan Bay and Irish Sea

Cardigan (Teifi Estuary) - St Dogmaels

Type:	concrete slipway
Suits:	craft up to 25'/7.6m LOA
Availability:	approx. 2 hours either side HW
Restrictions:	speed limit in certain areas: beware strong currents
Facilities:	parking for car and trailer, toilets and pub nearby
Dues:	none
Charge:	none
Directions:	from Cardigan follow B4546 through St Dogmaels: site is on west bank of Teifi Estuary
Waters accessed:	Teifi Estuary, Cardigan Bay and Irish Sea

Newport - Newport Sands
Tel: (01437) 764636 (Pembrokeshire Coast National Park)

Type:	launching over hard sandy beach
Suits:	small craft which can be manhandled and sailboards
Availability:	all states of tide
Restrictions:	8 knot speed limit in estuary and off beach: wind-surfers must keep clear of bathing areas
Facilities:	parking for car and trailer on site (c), toilets, Inshore Rescue Boat and Lifeguard
Dues:	none
Charge:	none at present

Directions:	from Newport take the coast road towards Moylgrove, turning left to beach after 2 miles
Waters accessed:	Newport Bay and Irish Sea

Newport - Parrog
Tel: (01437) 764636 (Pembrokeshire Coast National Park)

Type:	concrete slipway onto hard sand
Suits:	craft up to 20'/6.1m LOA and sailboards
Availability:	approx. 1½ hours either side HW
Restrictions:	8 knot speed limit in estuary: windsurfers must keep clear of bathing areas: access road is narrow
Facilities:	fuel nearby, parking for car and trailer and toilets on site
Dues:	none
Charge:	none
Directions:	from Fishguard follow A487 to Newport: take minor road north following signs to 'Parrog' for ½ mile: access to site is through car park
Waters accessed:	Newport Bay and Irish Sea

Dinas Head - Cwym Yr Eglwys
Tel: (01437) 764636 (Pembrokeshire Coast National Park)

Type:	concrete slipway onto sandy beach
Suits:	small craft which can be manhandled
Availability:	approx. 3 hours either side HW
Restrictions:	8 knot speed limit in bay: pwc and water-skiing prohibited; site has narrow access road with sharp bend and is very congested in summer; beware strong currents off Dinas Head
Facilities:	limited parking for car (c) but little space for trailers
Dues:	none
Charge:	none
Directions:	from Fishguard follow A487 north turn left onto minor road after Dinas Cross for 1 mile: site is on east side of Dinas Head
Waters accessed:	Newport Bay and Irish Sea

Dinas Head - Pwllgwaelod
Tel: (01437) 764636 (Pembrokeshire Coast National Park)

Type:	concrete slipway onto hard sand
Suits:	small craft, windsurfers and canoes
Availability:	all states of tide
Restrictions:	8 knots speed limit within 100m of shore: beware strong currents off Dinas Head
Facilities:	parking for car and trailer, toilets, restaurant all on site
Dues:	none
Charge:	none at present
Directions:	from Fishguard follow A487 north turning left onto minor road at Dinas Cross for 1 mile: site is on west side of Dinas Head
Waters accessed:	Fishguard Bay and Irish Sea

Fishguard - Lower Town

Tel: (01348) 873369/874726 - mobile (07775) 523846 (Harbour Master)

Type:	concrete slipway onto hard sand
Suits:	small craft, windsurfers and canoes
Availability:	all states of tide
Restrictions:	6 knot speed limit in harbour: no water-skiing; access to site is very narrow and larger craft should use Goodwick slipway (next entry)
Facilities:	parking for car and trailer, toilets
Dues:	none
Charge:	approx. £5 daily, £15 weekly or £40 monthly
Directions:	from Cardigan follow A487 south: site is at the end of the Quay
Waters accessed:	Fishguard Bay and Irish Sea

Fishguard (Ferry Port) - Goodwick Slipway

Tel: (01348) 404425 (Stena Line) or (01348) 874803 (Watersports Centre)

Type:	concrete slipway
Suits:	all craft
Availability:	approx. 2 hours either side HW
Restrictions:	speed limit in harbour: no water-skiing
Facilities:	fuel, parking for car and trailer, toilets, chandlery, watersports centre adjacent
Dues:	none known
Charge:	none
Directions:	from Cardigan follow A487 south: site is adjacent to car park and watersports centre on seafront
Waters accessed:	Fishguard Bay and Irish Sea

Porthgain

Tel: (01437) 764636 (Pembrokeshire Coast National Park)

Type:	concrete slipway into harbour
Suits:	powered craft up to 20'/6.1m LOA
Availability:	approx. 2 hours either side HW
Restrictions:	strong tide races just outside harbour make site unsuitable for dinghy sailing and water-skiing
Facilities:	fuel nearby (on A487), parking for car and trailer, toilets, pub and restaurant on site
Dues:	none
Charge:	ask at pub
Directions:	from Fishguard follow A487 south to Croesgoch: turn right onto minor road to Porthgain for 2 miles
Waters accessed:	Irish Sea

Abereiddy - Beach

Tel: (01437) 764636 (Pembrokeshire Coast National Park)

Type:	steep concrete slipway onto soft sand
Suits:	sailing dinghies, windsurfers and canoes
Availability:	approx. 4 hours either side HW
Restrictions:	8 knot speed limit within 100m of shore: trailers can get bogged down on the beach; there are rocky patches and strong currents offshore and large breakers build up on beach, especially in onshore winds
Facilities:	fuel nearby (on A487), parking for car and trailer on site, toilets
Dues:	none
Charge:	none
Directions:	from Fishguard follow A487 south through Croesgoch: turn right onto minor road signposted Abereiddy for 2 miles
Waters accessed:	Irish Sea

Porthclais - Porthclais Boat Owners Assoc. Slipway

Tel: (01437) 764636 (Pembrokeshire Coast National Park)

Type:	concrete slipway
Suits:	craft up to 25'/7.6m LOA
Availability:	approx. 2½ hours either side HW
Restrictions:	speed limit inshore: slipway may be obstructed by locked barrier out of season; access through St Davids is narrow and may be congested
Facilities:	fuel from garage (2 miles), parking for car nearby, and for trailer on site, toilets, other facilities in St Davids (1½ miles)
Dues:	none
Charge:	payable to Portclais Boat Owners Assoc.
Directions:	from Fishguard follow A487 south to St Davids then signs for Porthclais
Waters accessed:	St Brides Bay and Irish Sea

Solva - Solva Boat Owners Assoc. Slipway

Tel: (01437) 764636 (Pembrokeshire Coast National Park)

Type:	concrete slipways
Suits:	small craft only
Availability:	approx. 2-3 hours either side HW
Restrictions:	8 knot speed limit: no water-skiing: a very beautiful site which is often congested in summer
Facilities:	parking for car and trailer, toilets, pubs, shops and restaurant all on site
Dues:	none
Charge:	payable to Solva Boat Owners Assoc.
Directions:	from St Davids follow A487 east: site is on north shore of St Brides bay and access is through car park
Waters accessed:	St Brides Bay and Irish Sea

Nolton Haven

Type:	small ramp to top of shingle and sand beach
Suits:	small craft only
Availability:	approx. 3 hours either side HW
Restrictions:	8 knot speed limit inshore: site is exposed in westerlys
Facilities:	petrol nearby (Simpson Cross), parking for car on site and for trailer nearby, toilets, pub, restaurant
Dues:	none
Charge:	none
Directions:	from Haverfordwest follow A487 west: turn left following signs to Nolton Haven 1 mile after Simpsons Cross
Waters accessed:	St Brides Bay and Irish Sea

Broad Haven

Tel: (01437) 764551 (Pembrokeshire County Council)

Type:	shallow concrete ramp onto hard sand beach
Suits:	all craft
Availability:	all states of tide
Restrictions:	8 knot speed limit in bay: no pwc or water-skiing; vehicles are only allowed on beach to assist in launch and recovery but must then be removed; dangerous surf in westerly winds
Facilities:	fuel nearby, parking for car and trailer (c), toilets, pub and shops on site
Dues:	none
Charge:	none
Directions:	from Haverfordwest follow B4341 west
Waters accessed:	St Brides Bay and Irish Sea

Little Haven

Tel: (01437) 764551 (Pembrokeshire County Council)

Type:	shallow concrete ramp onto hard sand beach
Suits:	small craft
Availability:	all states of tide
Restrictions:	8 knot speed limit in bay: no pwc or water-skiing in bay; no vehicles allowed on beach; access roads to site are steep; **Note:** slipway must be kept clear at all times for use of Lifeboat
Facilities:	fuel nearby, parking for car and trailer (c), toilets and pub on site , chandlers, outboard repairs and diving supplies nearby
Dues:	none
Charge:	none
Directions:	from Haverfordwest follow B4327 west to Hasguard Cross and then signs to Little Haven
Waters accessed:	St Brides Bay and Irish Sea

Marloes - Martin's Haven

Tel: (01437) 764551 (Pembrokeshire County Council)

Type:	steep road onto shingle foreshore
Suits:	small craft
Availability:	approx. 2 hours either side HW
Restrictions:	8 knot speed limit in bay: site is adjacent Skomer Marine Nature Reserve where there are voluntary restrictions for craft; there are dangerous currents in Broad Sound; this is a difficult site
Facilities:	fuel nearby, limited parking for car and trailer (c) and toilets on site, chandlery, outboard repairs and diving supplies nearby
Dues:	none
Charge:	none
Directions:	from Haverfordwest follow B4327 west towards Dale turning north onto minor road to Marloes
Waters accessed:	St Brides Bay and Irish Sea

Dale (Milford Haven Waterway) - Dale Slipway

Tel: (01437) 764636 (Pembrokeshire Coast National Park)

Type:	shallow concrete ramp onto shingle/sand
Suits:	craft up to 18'/5.5m-20'/6.1m LOA
Availability:	at all states of tide
Restrictions:	8 knot speed limit in bay - no planing: this is a major windsurfing centre; pwc and water-skiing permitted outside bay; narrow access road and site can be congested in summer
Facilities:	fuel, parking for car and trailer (c), toilets, chandlery, outboard repairs, diving supplies, pubs and cafe all on site
Dues:	none
Charge:	none
Directions:	from Haverfordwest follow B4327 west or minor roads from Milford Haven
Waters accessed:	Milford Haven Waterway and Irish Sea

Gellyswick Bay (Milford Haven Waterway) - Slipway

Tel: (01437) 764636 (Pembrokeshire Coast National Park)

Type:	wide concrete slipway onto hard sand
Suits:	all craft up to 40'/12.2m LOA and 8'/2.4m draught
Availability:	all states of tide except LWS
Restrictions:	8 knot speed limit in bay: pwc and water-skiing permitted in designated areas; access is via a steep hill
Facilities:	fuel (1 mile), parking for car and trailer on site, toilets and all other facilities from boatyards and marinas nearby
Dues:	none
Charge:	none

Directions:	from Milford Haven, take road past Hakin to Hubberston, turning left opposite petrol station and following road to Gellyswick Bay: site is opposite Pembrokeshire Y.C. clubhouse
Waters accessed:	Milford Haven and Irish Sea

Milford Haven (Milford Haven Waterway) - Milford Marina, The Docks
Tel: (01646) 696312 (24 hour)

Type:	two steep concrete slipways
Suits:	all craft
Availability:	approx. 4 hours either side HW
Restrictions:	pwc and water-skiing permitted in designated areas
Facilities:	diesel on site, petrol nearby, parking for car and trailer, toilets, chandlery, outboard repairs, cranage, boat hoist all on site
Dues:	approx. £3
Charge:	no additional fee
Directions:	from Haverfordwest follow A478 to Milford Haven
Waters accessed:	Milford Haven Waterway and Irish Sea

Neyland (Milford Haven Waterway) - Promenade Slipway
Tel: (01437) 764636 (Pembokeshire Coast National Park))

Type:	concrete ramp
Suits:	all craft up to 18'/5.5m-20'/6.1m LOA
Availability:	all states of tide except LWS
Restrictions:	pwc and water-skiing permitted in designated areas: beware strong tidal currents and eddies; launching is difficult in south-westerly winds
Facilities:	parking for car and trailer on site, fuel and other facilities nearby
Dues:	none
Charge:	none
Directions:	from Haverfordwest follow A4076 then A477: site is on Promenade next to Neyland Y.C.
Waters accessed:	Milford Haven and Irish Sea

Neyland (Milford Haven Waterway) - Dale Sailing Co. Brunel Quay
Tel: (01646) 601636

Type:	launching by hoist into marina basin
Suits:	larger craft up to 35 ton
Availability:	during working hours by prior arrangement
Restrictions:	5 mph speed limit in marina entrance
Facilities:	diesel on site, petrol nearby, parking for car and trailer, chandlery, outboard repairs and all marina facilities on site, toilets nearby
Dues:	none
Charge:	approx. £45 each way
Directions:	from Haverfordwest follow A4076/A477 to Neyland and signs to marina
Waters accessed:	Milford Haven and Irish Sea

Llangwm (Daucleddau Estuary) - Black Tar Point
Tel: (01437) 764636 (Pembrokeshire Coast National Park)

Type:	concrete slipway
Suits:	all craft up to approx. 18'/5.5m LOA: no pwc
Availability:	approx. 5 hours either side HW
Restrictions:	slow speed in mooring area - no planing; access road is narrow in places; site is in heart of National Park - do not park on foreshore
Facilities:	fuel from garages nearby, limited parking for car and trailer and toilets on site, other facilities from Neyland or Pembroke Dock
Dues:	none
Charge:	none, but donations to Llangwm Boatowners Assoc. appreciated
Directions:	from Haverfordwest follow A4076 south turning left onto minor roads and following signs to Black Tar Point: site is about 5 miles south of Haverfordwest
Waters accessed:	Cleddau River, Milford Haven and Irish Sea

Haverfordwest (Daucleddau Estuary) - Old Quay, Quay Street
Tel: (01437) 764636 (Pembrokeshire Coast National Park)

Type:	very small narrow concrete ramp
Suits:	small powered craft and canoes only
Availability:	approx. 2 hours either side HW
Restrictions:	low speed: access to site is narrow and bridge down river prohibits craft with masts from launching
Facilities:	fuel in town, parking for car and trailer on site, other facilities from Neyland and Pembroke Dock
Dues:	none
Charge:	none
Directions:	from Carmarthen follow A40 west to Haverfordwest
Waters accessed:	Daucleddau Estuary and Milford Haven Waterway

Landshipping Ferry (Cleddau River) - Foreshore
Tel: (01437) 764636 (Pembrokeshire Coast National Park)

Type:	launching over hard mud/shingle foreshore
Suits:	sailing dinghies, small powered craft and canoes
Availability:	approx. 3 hours either side HW
Restrictions:	low speed - no planing: narrow access roads; site is in heart of National Park
Facilities:	very limited parking for car and trailer on site, toilets and pub nearby
Dues:	none
Charge:	none
Directions:	from Carmarthen follow A40 west to Canaston Bridge, turning left onto A4075 to Cross Hands; turn right onto minor roads to Landshipping
Waters accessed:	Cleddau River and Milford Haven Waterway

Lawrenny (Milford Haven Waterway) - Lawrenny Yacht Station
Tel: (01646) 651212/651439

Type:	shallow concrete ramp
Suits:	all craft
Availability:	all states of tide
Restrictions:	4 mph speed limit in moorings
Facilities:	fuel, parking for car and trailer, toilets and showers, chandlery, outboard repairs and other facilities
Dues:	none
Charge:	approx. £3
Directions:	from Carmarthen follow A40 and A477 west to Carew, turning right onto A4075 to Cresselly then following signposted minor roads
Waters accessed:	Cleddau River, Milford Haven Waterway and Irish Sea

Hobbs Point (Milford Haven Waterway) - Pier Road Slipway
Tel: (01646) 696100 (Milford Haven Port Authority)

Type:	broad, but steep, concrete slipway with drop at end at LWS
Suits:	all craft
Availability:	approx. 5 hours either side HW
Restrictions:	speed limit: water-skiing and pwc permitted in designated areas nearby; beware strong currents and eddies: site is used by Pembroke Haven Y.C.
Facilities:	fuel nearby, very limited parking for car and trailer, toilets, chandlery, diving supplies and outboard repairs all on site
Dues:	none
Charge:	none
Directions:	follow A477 into Pembroke Dock going down Pier Rd past Kwik Save supermarket to Hobbs Point
Waters accessed:	Milford Haven Waterway and Irish Sea

Pembroke Dock (Milford Haven Waterway) - Front Street
Tel: (01646) 696100 (Milford Haven Port Authority)

Type:	shallow concrete slipway which tends to silt up at bottom end
Suits:	all craft
Availability:	approx. 5 hours either side HW
Restrictions:	slow speed in moorings: pwc and water-skiing permitted in designated areas nearby; site is used by Pembroke Haven Motor Boat Club
Facilities:	fuel nearby, parking for car and trailer on site, toilets and other facilities available nearby, museum adjacent
Dues:	none
Charge:	none
Directions:	follow A477 into Pembroke Dock, turning into Criterion Way and then Front St.: site is at corner of Front St and Commercial Rd
Waters accessed:	Milford Haven Waterway and Irish Sea

Pembroke - Castle Pond
Tel: (01646) 694011 (Pembrokeshire County Council)

Type:	concrete slipway
Suits:	dinghies and canoes
Availability:	0900-1700 daily: check for availability with Pembrokeshire Watersports School (01646) 622013
Restrictions:	on certain tides the pond is completely emptied; passage of boats into the Pembroke River is allowed approx. 1 hour either side HW
Facilities:	fuel nearby, limited parking for car and trailer on site (c), toilets on site, cafe and shops nearby
Dues:	none
Charge:	none
Directions:	turn off A4139 near Waterman's Arms into small public car park adjacent to Pembroke Castle
Waters accessed:	Castle Pond is above the Pembroke Barrage

Angle (Milford Haven Waterway) - Angle Bay
Tel: (01437) 764636 (Pembrokeshire Coast National Park))

Type:	launching over shingle foreshore
Suits:	craft up to 21'/6.4m LOA
Availability:	approx. 3 hours either side HW
Restrictions:	water-skiing permitted in designated areas nearby: narrow access road to site; area is part of National Park
Facilities:	fuel nearby, very limited parking for car and trailer, pub and toilets nearby, other facilities available from Pembroke Dock
Dues:	none
Charge:	none
Directions:	from Pembroke follow B4320 to Angle; turn right in village following signs to RNLI Lifeboat
Waters accessed:	Milford Haven Waterway and Irish Sea

Freshwater East
Tel: (01437) 764636 (Pembrokeshire Coast National Park)

Type:	steep concrete slipway onto sandy beach which is soft in places
Suits:	small craft at all times; larger craft need 4-wheel drive vehicle to tow across beach
Availability:	all states of tide
Restrictions:	navigate with due care and attention: access road is narrow; no parking on beach
Facilities:	limited parking for car and trailer nearby (c), toilets
Dues:	none
Charge:	none
Directions:	from Pembroke follow A4139 east to Lamphey; turn right onto B4584 and follow signs
Waters accessed:	Carmarthen Bay

Lydstep Haven - Lydstep Beach Holiday Resort

Tel: (01834) 871871

Type:	steep concrete slipway onto hard sandy beach
Suits:	all craft
Availability:	all states of tide 0900-1800
Restrictions:	speed limit; water-skiing permitted outside buoys off beach; evidence of insurance including 3rd party cover must be produced
Facilities:	limited parking for car and trailer (c), accommodation and toilets on site
Dues:	none
Charge:	approx. £30 a day / £80 a week for non-residents
Directions:	from Tenby follow A4139 west towards Pembroke and follow signs to Lydstep Haven
Waters accessed:	Carmarthen Bay

Tenby - Harbour Slipway

Tel: (01834) 842717 or (07977) 099471 (Harbour Office, Castle Square)

Type:	steep concrete slipway onto hard sand foreshore
Suits:	craft up to 16'/4.9m LOA except pwc
Availability:	approx. 2½ hours either side HW during daylight hours by arrangement
Restrictions:	3 knot speed limit in Inner Harbour, 10 knots in Outer Harbour: water-skiing permitted in designated area but pwc prohibited: site is very congested in summer and access is via very narrow and busy town centre roads with steep road into basin
Facilities:	fuel in town, very limited parking for car and trailer (c), toilets, diving supplies and outboard repairs, cafes and restaurants on site, limited chandlery nearby
Dues:	approx. £2 (sailing craft) or £3 (motor craft)
Charge:	no additional fee
Directions:	from Carmarthen follow A40/A477/A478 to Tenby: turn off along Narberth Rd to North Beach, going through Tudor Sq. (town centre) to harbour: site is adjacent to Tenby S.C.
Waters accessed:	Carmarthen Bay

Saundersfoot - Harbour Slipway

Tel: (01834) 812094 (Harbour Office)

Type:	concrete slipway onto hard sand
Suits:	all craft
Availability:	approx. 2-2½ hours either side HW or at all states of tide over sand for dinghies
Restrictions:	3 knot speed limit in harbour and within 250m of shore: water-skiing permitted in designated area outside this: certificate of insurance cover required: site can be congested in summer
Facilities:	fuel nearby, parking for car and trailer, toilets, chandlery nearby

Dues:	approx. £5.50 inc. parking for car and trailer
Charge:	no additional charge
Directions:	from Carmarthen follow A40/A477/A478 to Pentlepoir: turn left onto B4316 to Saundersfoot
Waters accessed:	Carmarthen Bay

Amroth - Amroth Beach

Type:	steep L-shaped concrete slipway
Suits:	craft up to approx.16'/4.9m LOA
Availability:	approx. 1 hour either side HW or across beach at other times
Restrictions:	all vessels to operate 500m offshore: no vehicles or trailers to remain on beach
Facilities:	parking for car and trailer and toilets nearby
Dues:	none
Charge:	none
Directions:	from Carmarthen follow A40/A477 to Llanteg: turn left onto minor roads to Amroth village and follow road along coast to Amroth Castle: site is adjacent Amroth Castle Caravan Park
Waters accessed:	Carmarthen Bay

Laugharne (Taf Estuary) - Beach

Type:	launching over hard shingle beach
Suits:	small craft only
Availability:	approx. 2 hours either side HW
Restrictions:	none known
Facilities:	fuel in village, parking for car and trailer, toilets
Dues:	none
Charge:	none
Directions:	from Carmarthen follow A40 to St Clears turning left onto A4066: site is by Castle
Waters accessed:	Taf Estuary and Carmarthen Bay

Llangain (River Towy) - Towy Boat Club, Llanstephan Road

Type:	launching over shingle
Suits:	small craft only
Availability:	approx. 2 hours either side HW
Restrictions:	5 knot speed limit
Facilities:	parking for car and trailer
Dues:	none
Charge:	yes
Directions:	from Carmarthen follow B4312 south
Waters accessed:	River Towy and Carmarthen Bay

Carmarthen (River Towy) - The Quay (Carmarthen Boat Club)

Type:	steep concrete slipway
Suits:	small powered craft only
Availability:	approx. 2 hours either side HW
Restrictions:	5 knot speed limit: water-skiing permitted in designated area; headroom restricted down river
Facilities:	fuel from garage nearby, parking for car and trailer (c)
Dues:	none
Charge:	yes
Directions:	site is off A40
Waters accessed:	River Towy and Carmarthen Bay

Ferryside (River Towy) - River Towy Yacht Club, The Foreshore
Tel: (01267) 267366

Type:	shallow concrete slipway
Suits:	all craft
Availability:	approx. 2½ hours either side HW with permission
Restrictions:	5 knot speed limit in moorings: water-skiing permitted in designated area; very long craft may have problems grounding over railway crossing; best site in area
Facilities:	parking for car and trailer (c), toilets and showers on site; members have use of tractor
Dues:	none
Charge:	approx. £5 (recoverable on joining club)
Directions:	from Carmarthen follow A48/A484 south: turn off at LLandyfaelog and follow signs; site is across level crossing in centre of Ferryside
Waters accessed:	River Towy and Carmarthen Bay

Kidwelly (River Gwendraeth) - Quay

Type:	concrete slipway
Suits:	all craft
Availability:	approx. 2 hours either side HW
Restrictions:	none known
Facilities:	fuel in village, parking for car and trailer
Dues:	none
Charge:	none
Directions:	from Carmarthen follow A48/A484 south: site is 1 mile SW of Kidwelly and access is via Station Rd and over railway line
Waters accessed:	River Gwendraeth and Carmarthen Bay

Burry Port (Burry Inlet) - Harbour Slipway
Tel: (01554) 834315 (Harbour Master)

Type:	four concrete slipways
Suits:	all craft
Availability:	approx. 3 hours either side HW
Restrictions:	3 knot speed limit within harbour limits: water-skiing permitted in Burry Inlet: the bar at the entrance is dangerous in strong westerly winds; major changes are to be made to this site - please contact (01554) 777744 or (01267) 234567 for further details
Facilities:	fuel nearby, parking for car and trailer on site, toilets, chandlery and repairs all available on site
Dues:	none
Charge:	none**Directions:** turn off M4 at junction 48, taking the A4138 to Llanelli and then A484 to Burry Port
Waters accessed:	Burry Inlet, River Loughor and Carmarthen Bay

Llanelli (Burry Inlet)- Slipway

Type:	concrete slipway
Suits:	all craft
Availability:	all states of tide
Restrictions:	speed limit: water-skiing permitted in Burry Inlet; major changes are to be made to Burry Inlet - please contact (01554) 777744 or (01267) 234567 for further details
Facilities:	fuel (1/4 mile), parking for car and trailer
Dues:	none
Charge:	none
Directions:	turn off M4 at junction 48, taking the A4138 to Llanelli: site is 1/2 mile south of town centre and access is via Queen Victoria Rd and Cambrian St, turning right along track across open ground
Waters accessed:	Burry Inlet, River Loughor and Carmarthen Bay

Swansea - Port Eynon Bay
Tel: (01792) 635436 (City and County of Swansea)

Type:	concrete road onto beach
Suits:	small craft: 4-wheel drive vehicle recommended
Availability:	at most states of tide across beach
Restrictions:	4 knot speed limit: narrow access lane; all powered craft over 15hp must be registered (c)
Facilities:	parking for car and trailer (c) and toilets on site
Dues:	registration fee approx. £3 or £2 if member of local club
Charge:	none
Directions:	follow A4118 west from Swansea to south shore of Gower Peninsula
Waters accessed:	Bristol Channel

Mumbles, Swansea - Knab Rock and Southend Boat Parks
Tel: (01792) 635436 (City and County of Swansea)

Type:	(1) steep concrete ramp
	(2) two shallow concrete ramps onto pebbles
Suits:	all craft
Availability:	approx. 3-4 hours either side HW
Restrictions:	4 knot speed limit in moorings: one slipway has a barrier and is for the use of non-powered craft only; all powered craft over 15hp must be registered (c)
Facilities:	fuel (1 mile), parking for car and trailer (c) and toilets on site, chandlery and other facilities in Swansea
Dues:	registration fee approx. £3 or £2 if member of local club
Charge:	approx. £4.25 inc. parking
Directions:	from Swansea follow A4067 west to Mumbles: site is opposite Mumbles Y.C.
Waters accessed:	Swansea Bay

Swansea - Swansea Yacht and Sub-Aqua Club, Pocketts Wharf
Tel: (01792) 469084 mon-fri 0930-1430 or (01792) 654863 at weekends

Type:	concrete slipway
Suits:	all craft except ski-boats and pwc
Availability:	at all times by arrangement with Club Bosun or Secretary
Restrictions:	4 knot speed limit: water-skiing and pwc prohibited
Facilities:	fuel nearby, parking for car nearby and for trailer on site, toilets and showers in clubhouse, chandlery and repairs nearby
Dues:	none
Charge:	approx. £25 for non-members
Directions:	leave M4 at junction 47 taking A483 to Swansea: site adjoins East Burrows Rd
Waters accessed:	River Tawe and Swansea Bay (via lock)

Swansea - Swansea Marina, Lockside
Tel: (01792) 470310

Type:	launching by marine travel hoist only into locked marina basin
Suits:	larger craft
Availability:	0800-1400 by prior arrangement
Restrictions:	4 knot speed limit: lock gates open for $4\frac{1}{2}$ hours either side HW
Facilities:	diesel on site, petrol nearby, parking for car and trailer, toilets, chandlery and outboard repairs all available on site
Dues:	none
Charge:	approx. £70.50
Directions:	leave M4 at junction 47 and take A483 to Swansea, then A4067 and follow signs to marina
Waters accessed:	Swansea Bay (via lock) and Bristol Channel

Port Talbot - Aberavon Beach

Type:	two concrete slipways onto beach
Suits:	craft up to 20'/6.1m LOA
Availability:	all states of tide
Restrictions:	speed limit inshore
Facilities:	fuel, parking for car and trailer, toilets
Dues:	none
Charge:	none
Directions:	leave M4 at junction 41 and follow signs
Waters accessed:	Swansea Bay and Bristol Channel

Porthcawl - Harbour Slipway

Tel: (01656) 782756

Type:	steep concrete ramp
Suits:	small powered craft
Availability:	approx. 3 hours either side HW
Restrictions:	3 knot speed limit: access to slipway has low overhead telephone cables; priority must be given to RNLI Lifeboat; site is exposed and there are very strong currents
Facilities:	fuel nearby, parking for car and trailer on site, toilets nearby
Dues:	none
Charge:	approx. £3
Directions:	leave M4 at junction 37 taking A4229 and following signs to seafront
Waters accessed:	Bristol Channel

Barry - Watch Tower Bay, The Knap

Tel: (01446) 709569

Type:	concrete slipway
Suits:	small craft except pwc
Availability:	approx. 3 hours either side HW
Restrictions:	speed limit near beach: pwc prohibited; vehicles prohibited from slipway; strong currents inshore
Facilities:	parking for car nearby, limited space for trailers on site, toilets nearby
Dues:	none
Charge:	annual permit required (£5, numbers limited)
Directions:	leave M4 at junction 33 and take A4232 /A4050 south to Barry following signs to 'The Knap'
Waters accessed:	Severn Estuary and Bristol Channel

Sully - Council Slipway, Hayes Road

Tel: (01446) 709569

Type:	shallow concrete ramp
Suits:	small saling and powered craft
Availability:	approx. 3½ hours either side HW

Restrictions:	speed limit inshore: access has narrow (8'/2.4m) gateway; strong current inshore; site unsafe in winds over force 4 from SE to SW
Facilities:	fuel nearby, parking for car and trailer on site
Dues:	none
Charge:	none
Directions:	leave M4 at junction 33 taking A4232 /A4050 south to Barry following signs to Barry Dock: at roundabout at link road take turning for Sully and then take 2nd left at next roundabout: site is behind municipal amenity waste site
Waters accessed:	Severn Estuary and Bristol Channel

Penarth - Northern Slipway, The Esplanade
Tel: (01446) 709569 or 029 20708212 May - Sept

Type:	narrow and steep concrete slipway
Suits:	small craft
Availability:	approx. 3 hours either side HW
Restrictions:	8 knot speed limit inshore
Facilities:	fuel nearby, parking for car and trailer (c) and toilets on site
Dues:	none
Charge:	annual permit required: residents £15, non-residents £25
Directions:	leave M4 at junction 33 taking A4232 to Penarth and following signs through town to seafront: site is situated under the multi-storey car park
Waters accessed:	Severn Estuary and Bristol Channel

Penarth - Southern Slipway
Tel: (01446) 709569 or 029 20708212 May - Sept

Type:	concrete slipway with sharp bend
Suits:	sailing craft and small powered craft (under 25hp): no pwc
Availability:	approx. 3 hours either side HW
Restrictions:	speed limit: powered craft over 25hp and pwc prohibited
Facilities:	fuel nearby, parking for car and trailer nearby, toilets nearby
Dues:	none
Charge:	annual permit required: residents £15, non-residents £25
Directions:	leave M4 at junction 33 taking A4232 to Penarth and following signs through town to seafront: site is in front of Y.C.
Waters accessed:	Severn Estuary and Bristol Channel

Penarth - Penarth Marina

Tel: 029 20705021

Type:	launching for boats up to 20 tons by travel hoist into locked marina basin
Suits:	larger craft
Availability:	0900-1730 by prior arrangement
Restrictions:	speed limit in bay
Facilities:	fuel, parking for car and trailer (c), toilets, chandlery, outboard repairs, berths, storage ashore and all marina facilities
Dues:	none
Charge:	approx. £8.50 per metre each way
Directions:	leave M4 at junction 32 following signs to 'Cardiff Bay' and Penarth and follow signs to marina
Waters accessed:	Cardiff Bay and Bristol Channel via lock

Rudyard, Staffs - Rudyard Lake

Tel: (01538) 306280 (Information Centre)

Type:	concrete slipway
Suits:	sailing craft up to 28'/8.5m LOA
Availability:	during daylight hours
Restrictions:	powered craft prohibited: narrow access road
Facilities:	parking for car and trailer (c) and toilets on site
Dues:	none
Charge:	approx. £4.50
Directions:	from Leek follow A523 north for 3 miles, turning left to Rudyard: at roundabout turn right and immediately right again into Lake Rd: entrance is 250m on right
Waters accessed:	Rudyard Lake only

INDEX